HEALTH — A SURPRISING JOY

Health and the Christian Church

Roy Billington

CMS

Church Missionary Society
157 Waterloo Road, London SE1 8UU
1976

ISBN No. 0 900287 28 4

Printed by Bocardo & Church Army Press Ltd., Cowley, Oxford, England

Health is a surprising joy

Dr. Robert Lambourne

To Dora

CONTENTS

FOREWORD

One of our local church house groups meets regularly in our house. One evening recently we were conscious that our times of Bible Study have been drawing us more deeply together and also getting us ready to go out more into the neighbourhood. An old people's home in the neighbouring road looked like being the starting point. I read some passages from this exciting and encouraging book to the group; in particular, the description of the ways in which old people had been brought to life and had flowered, finding their own gifts, in response to a new kind of caring. The group was quite fired by this and encouraged to feel its own potential.

Throughout the world at this time, Christians are making similar discoveries of their new corporate potential in "the Body of Christ". This kind of discovery brings with it an exhilarating change in our whole understanding of Christian mission. The hospital and the clinic, like the school or the agricultural centre or industrial mission, have traditionally come into being separated from each other and from worshipping congregations and, like the latter, run by experts. Now healing, like learning and rural and urban development, is becoming a vital aspect of congregational life in which every member has a ministry. "Health" embraces all these activities and is seen not just as a physical or mental state but supremely as a quality of relationships. And evangelism is the cutting edge of the Christian community.

This picture of health and healing is a fulfilment of an insight that was always present in traditional cultures, and that seems even harder to develop further in the West than it does in the Third World. Christians in the West can come to it only if they find themselves in the world-wide Body of Christ, just as they rediscover their corporate life locally. Then, if people and ideas and experiences go to and fro in the world, we can all learn afresh from each other what health and community mean. And, as this happens, we shall realize more and more that the healing in the world-wide Body depends a good deal on how we in the West rise to our terrible responsibilities. We deprive so many other people in the world of the health that is their right just because we depend for our own material wellbeing on their poverty.

But if health is essentially a product of true community, world-wide and local, without which our Gospel will not be fully conveyed, then our tiny little local efforts everywhere are, as Roy Billington says, significant in Hakan Hellberg's sense. Each person, each little group can "make a sign" that will point to new life. Roy himself has been just such a sign to many both in Uganda and more recently in his world-wide responsibilities as Medical Secretary of CMS. In his characteristically gentle, humble way, and yet with firm and clear persistence, he has been summoning us all to this new vision of health and the healing aspects of the whole community's life.

This vision is, alas, still all too rare, especially in the West. The great value of this book is that it expresses all that its author has been saying to us in his own life in a stimulating and compelling way, drawing for its illustrations upon a world-wide experience. I believe and hope it will inspire many more people not only to come to a wider understanding of health, but also to join in putting that understanding into practice.

SIMON BARRINGTON-WARD

PREFACE

This is a short book on developing patterns of "medical missions" or, more correctly, on Christian health care or church-related health care, particularly in the Third World.

Such Christian medical work is going through great changes today, and I am anxious to see first, how it can remain distinctively Christian, using many of the emphases of the World Health Organization or other health planners, but making these part of the total witness of the Christian congregation to the love and power of Christ.

Second, how it can form a natural part of the life of a Christian community, integrated with other sides of that life, such as farming, craft employment and education, and at the same time reach out from the community to neighbours of other faiths.

And third, how it can become a type of health care in which non-medical Christians can take a personal and effective share.

I begin with some of the questions for which I need an answer, and then look for these answers, first in the Bible, and then in the stimulating writings of Christian medical thinkers.

From these a pattern emerges which underlines the importance of the family as the God-given unit on which society is built. Health care begins with the family. And then comes the community, rural or urban, with its varied needs, the community in which health interacts with other sides of life.

The remarkable achievements of China are studied, and subsequent chapters deal with the notable contributions that a hospital makes in any neighbourhood; with relevant health training at different levels; and with the great gains that come when different health enterprises plan and work together.

The rest of the book is concerned with warm acceptance of those who are in danger of rejection by society; with the place of prayer in healing; the need to understand and appreciate traditional medicine in its varied forms; and Christian responsibility to promote justice and constructive social action as part of a concern for the health of others.

In what I have written I have been very conscious of many shortcomings and much ignorance, particularly in the fields of "spiritual healing" and anthropology. But I have nevertheless realized that some of the principles which we in the West are trying to learn, such as establishing a close link between religion and medicine, or building up a strong caring community, or seeing health as only one part of many-sided social living, have been part of the fabric of life in developing countries for years without number. If we have something to offer in the field of health, we have also very much to receive.

I owe much to the Christian Medical Commission for its stimulating writings, and I quote from these frequently. I am very grateful to all those who have published accounts of pioneer ventures which I have been able to describe.

In chapter 3 I make use of diagrams adapted from the writings of Robert Lambourne, whose far-sighted thinking has put us all in his debt.

Some of the diagrams also appear in Michael Wilson's excellent book *Health is for People*. My draft manuscript was actually completed before his book appeared. I am sure he will understand that I was not intending to copy his approach; we were in fact drawing our ideas from the same spring.

I deeply appreciate Canon Simon Barrington-Ward's generous foreword, and his close interest in richer community living. And I indeed thank my kind typists, Marian Boulton, Susan Gooday and Joan Petch.

ROY BILLINGTON

Note: Biblical references are from the Revised Standard Version unless otherwise stated.
Where costs of treatment, education etc. are quoted, an exchange rate of £1 = US $2.00 is used.

Chapter 1

ASKING MYSELF QUESTIONS

"It very soon became evident," wrote Albert Cook, pioneer missionary, in 1897, "that Uganda with its little-known diseases was a professional man's paradise. The range of surgical, medical, gynaecological and obstetric cases was immense, and work in every specialty lay open to the keen researcher."[1]

Somehow the issues seem to have been so much simpler when viewed by the gifted medical missionaries of those days. They went out with the love of Christ in their hearts and their western medical training in their brains and fingertips, to preach and to heal. Their skill, particularly surgical skill and ability to deal with difficult childbirth, quickly won them many friends who were ready to listen to the Gospel which they taught.

They built their hospitals and trained their staff, perhaps founding nursing schools and even medical colleges. Many a time the introduction of modern medical care over wide areas was entirely due to their efforts.

Today more than three thousand Christian medical institutions in developing countries are the legacy of their devotion, skill and love, and in some countries such as Tanzania and Malawi, 40% of all hospital beds have been provided by church hospitals.[2]

This is a noble record indeed, and something for which to be deeply thankful to God. But times change so fast that now there are many questions that press upon us, concerning the way that Christian health care should be carried out in today's world.

I had the great privilege of working in Albert Cook's own hospital, with many living memories of him and his achievements. But as time went by, I became more and more concerned to find an answer to such questions as, how can this great tradition of unselfish practical caring for others be adapted to present-day needs? What is the place of Christian concern for health in the life of the Church now? What changes ought we to be looking for?

How to meet the cost?

For a start, I couldn't forget that hospital work involved so much expense. This was not easily avoided, because trained staff were rightly paid at the accepted salary scales for the country. As a result however, fees charged to patients kept rising until a man could easily be asked to pay a day's wages in order to see the doctor and receive treatment, or a month's earnings to cover the cost of a stay in the wards.

Such charges were necessary to balance the budget and keep the hospital going, and indeed they did no more than meet a part of the actual cost of care. Patients certainly paid these charges (with generous Government grants making up the balance needed) but those who did so tended to be the better-off members of the community. Really poor people could not manage them.

It is true that in Uganda, as in Britain, Government hospitals provide free treatment. But the pressure on them was almost overwhelming at times. And it was painful to reflect that the church-related hospital could not afford to do more for the poorest and most needy in and around the city.

Small children were a particular problem. We wanted them to attend regularly at the "under-fives" clinic, but mothers could only afford to pay very little. So a mere token charge was made in this clinic, and hospital funds paid the rest.

Appropriate care

We had a tradition that a doctor saw every out-patient, at least on the first attendance—the "one-to-one" standard of care of British medicine. But eventually we realized that this was a waste of scarce doctors' time, and more and more of this work was delegated to others. Pregnant women and small children were almost all seen by midwives and nurses anyway.

Professor George Gale, one-time chairman of our Board of Governors, used to say "a hospital should make a big difference to the health of the community immediately around it," but this did not seem to be true in our case. So we hired two houses near a very crowded "shanty" area a mile away, in order that mothers could come there to have their babies, and then be taken home after 24 hours and visited during the following week. This worked well but had to be modified when rents were put up. As regards the actual community close to the hospital, I was conscious that indeed more could have been done.

Priorities in health

The years since I qualified as a doctor have witnessed the biggest advances in methods of preventing and treating disease that medical history has ever known, and it was thrilling to use the new tools of therapy one after another as they reached us in Africa.

But there were many frustrations. An elderly lady came into hospital bled white, as her tongue and eyelids showed, from hookworm anaemia. Blood transfusion and treatment for the worms soon put her right. But what could stop her being reinfected almost at once from the worms in the soil round her house, and then coming back in six months as pale as ever? Could we not do more for her than periodically resuscitate her in this way?

And small children suffered so much from preventable disease. Lack of enough protein and calories in their food caused kwashiorkor or "red boy", the West African name for the effect of malnutrition on a toddler, giving him reddish hair and a swollen body. Such children had a lowered resistance to infection and would quickly die from an attack of measles. Yet the country was most fertile and could easily grow all kinds of food.

Family health clinics were developed in the hospital and two or three villages, and demonstration food plots started. But were we stressing prevention and health education enough and doing all this in the right way?

Working to a plan

I often thought about the "end-point" of our work. What was our goal? When I talked to others about this, it was difficult to get a satisfactory answer. Perhaps the Government would take over church hospitals one day, they said, and that would be the end of the chapter.

Well, that was fine in a way: the hospitals would go on serving the country still. And indeed the Church could not begin to support such institutions from its own resources. But would nothing be left in the way of continued practical caring by the church? Would all this medical work just be a notable stage in the growth of the church and no more?

I knew that Christians had great resources to share, if not of money then of time and effort and compassion. How could these be used in ways which would witness to the love of Christ without great technical skill or long training being necessary, and with little or no expense?

Traditional medicine

I knew that nearly every patient, except the most consistent Christians, would use traditional remedies in times of sickness. But I understood so little about African concepts of health, disease and healing, to my shame. Kofi Appiah-Kubi has written very truthfully "It could be argued that the Church, through her various mission hospitals, has achieved a great deal in alleviating the physical sickness of the African Christian. But unfortunately this was done without any serious consideration of the people's own conception of the world in which they live and of the forces operating in it (the people's world-view), a conception which undoubtedly influences or determines their understanding of health and disease.

. . . "The Church must reconsider her healing ministry in Africa," he concludes, "in the light of the African world view"[3] . . . How was this understanding to be gained? It obviously called for much patient listening and willingness to learn.

Were we too materialistic?

In our medical work we wanted to put Jesus first. Every day the good news of His love was explained in wards and out-patients: patients were prayed with before operations, and at their bedsides: and we asked God to guide us in what we did.

But did our western scientific medical approach fit in adequately to a comprehensive view of man as a whole being? Africans, as Appiah-Kubi says again, make no distinction between religion and medicine in traditional thought. And indigenous African Christian churches believe in total personal healing, spiritual, psychological and physical, as being the gift of God.

Should we have prayed more specifically with our patients and their friends, praised God more for recoveries, and blurred the distinction between prayer and medicine as agents of healing?

In the right place?

In Uganda's Independence Year 1962 the big new University hospital of 800 beds was opened only three miles or so from where we worked. Were we still needed in the same city when rural areas had so little care?

We reflected that our training of nurses and midwives was of the greatest importance, and this was perhaps the chief reason why our work continued in the same place. But even about this training I could not help wondering sometimes.

It took 3 years to train a nurse at enrolled level, an additional year for her to become a nurse-midwife, and a further year again to qualify as that most valuable person, an assistant health visitor (or assistant public health nurse). Was all this length of training really needed to produce an all-round nurse at basic level?

Some of us met at the chief nursing training school, and revived plans for training a truly "comprehensive" nurse, who could become competent in hospital nursing, midwifery, psychiatry, and public health, all in under three years, as has indeed been achieved in other countries. She would have been so useful!—able to fit in anywhere. But the time was not favourable for such an advance, and the project was shelved again.

As we were in the city then, we thought of our responsibilities for our fellow citizens. Representatives of the four hospitals—one belonging to the medical school and three church-related—met to plan a City Health scheme, in order that a child leaving any hospital could go to the clinic nearest to where he lived and be sure of continuity of care. But again a sudden shortage of money and trained staff halted the plans and they were not revived.

The big enemies to health

When I left Uganda in 1973 to work at CMS headquarters in London, I was soon able to travel in Asia to see Christian medical work there. I was deeply impressed to learn afresh that on a world scale the greatest threats to health are not conditions for which a hospital is needed, and even a doctor would only play a minor part in dealing with them.

The first of these burdens is malnutrition. I learnt that 60% of the population in less developed countries is malnourished or badly fed, that is to say their food may be reasonable in amount, but it lacks certain constituents, such as good-quality protein, which are essential for health. And 20% are undernourished, receiving much less food than is necessary.[4] Malnutrition lowers resistance to infection, indirectly causing thousands of deaths daily. And in parts of Africa and India such as the Sahel or Maharastra, famine is an ever-present danger. Malnutrition is perhaps, after poverty, the second most important health problem in many parts of the world.

I saw, closely linked with this grave handicap, the crushing weight of preventable disease in developing countries. 40% of all deaths in the Third World occur in children under 5, from a combination of malnutrition, diseases caused by parasites, diarrhoea leading to dehydration, and other infections such as pneumonia. In Britain only 3% of all deaths take place in this age group.[5] Virtually all these conditions are preventable. But without an adequate programme to combat them, the deaths of toddlers may be fifty times commoner in Africa than in Europe—as was seen in Senegal in 1960.[6]

The third major enemy to health that I met everywhere was population pressure. The figures have been quoted so often that we hardly take them in. A world population of possibly more than six thousand millions is forecast for 2000 AD—having doubled itself in the 35 years from 1965 to the end of the century—with the fastest increase taking place in the poorest continents.[7]

The results of this population explosion are mounting pressure on world food supplies, large scale unemployment, and the seeming impossibility of ever providing enough schools and dispensaries for the needs of young children in particular.

And yet, surprisingly, each of these great threats to health, malnutrition, widespread preventable disease, and rapid population growth were brought under control in Europe during the nineteenth and early twentieth centuries without being directly attacked. The death rate fell steadily during that time, beginning before Pasteur had discovered the part that bacteria played in causing disease, and 50 or more years before Ehrlich had found the first specific drug which could cure infection.

As the death-rate from tuberculosis and the common infections of childhood came down, so the birth-rate began—after an interval—to fall likewise, until today the birth-rate in Europe is a quarter of that in South America. And all the time the level of nutrition of the population has been rising.

This story of steadily improved health was not, however, the result of better medical care. Smallpox was the only infection which doctors could prevent, and diseases for which specific cure existed were rare indeed.[8] It was greater prosperity, bringing better distribution of wealth, which saved lives and brought improved well-being.

And this improved standard of living is arguably the greatest need in world health today. Malnutrition is due largely to poverty, preventable diseases become widespread and dangerous because of poverty, and parents living in poverty need to have many children in order to be sure that some will survive. A more equitable spread of wealth, combined indeed with medical care and education in order to change human behaviour, would revolutionize the health picture of the world.[9] Without such a redistribution of world resources the outlook is bleak indeed.

As Peter Adamson says, we must solve the wealth problem in order to solve the food problem. And this of course is a political matter, which is dealt with in a later chapter.[10]

As I think about this I ask myself what should be the principles, the priorities, of Christian health workers in developing countries? Before trying to find an answer let me quote what John Bryant says about medical missionaries like myself.

"They are working in programmes of limited effectiveness," he comments trenchantly. "Usually they are engaged in curative work, which may often mean the treatment of symptoms only. Where those who come for treatment return to the same bad environment, no lasting benefit is received. The patterns of western medicine are too individualistic and therefore inappropriate," he continues. "Christian medical effort is often unrelated to any comprehensive programme. Efforts at prevention of disease are not co-ordinated. The educational schemes undertaken are complex and expensive, but of limited relevance."

In sum, he has the impression of enormous amounts of unavailing effort, in which diligence and dedication do not make up for the lack of critical assessment.[11]

Medical missionaries, together with other health professionals in developing countries, need to evaluate their work more fully. They should have clear goals, says Bryant; they should be adaptable, they should study the relation of agriculture, education and economics to their work. They should use plenty of common sense, and study alternative approaches to their task of bringing better health to man.[12]

After all, health, as Pascal de Pury says, is almost the same as happiness—certainly it is a part of happiness. The rest of this book will be devoted to considering how this stock of happiness can be increased more and more.[13]

1. Cook, A. R. *Uganda Memories*, Kampala, 1945.
2. Bryant, John. *Health and the Developing World,* Cornell, Ithaca N.Y., 1969, p. 304.
3. Appiah-Kubi, Kofi. *Ecumenical Review,* 1975, 27, 230.
4. *Medical Care in Developing Countries*, Office of Health Economics, London, 1972, p. 16.
5. ibid p. 18.
6. Bryant, John. op cit p. 36.
7. *Comment* no. 20, July 1974. Catholic Institute of International Relations, 41 Holland Park, London W.11.
8. *Medical Care in Developing Countries*, op cit pp. 3–4.
9. Smith, Tony. *The Times*, December 4 1974.
10. Adamson, Peter. *New Internationalist*, April 1975.
11. Bryant, John. op cit p. 321.
12. ibid p. 111.
13. de Pury, Pascal. *Rural Life*, 1974, **19**, 3.

Chapter 2

GOD'S PLAN FOR HEALTH AND HAPPINESS

To quote Pascal de Pury again, he sees health as a state of physical, mental and spiritual wellbeing, in which man is at home in his society, his culture and his environment, and has his heart full of love to God and to his neighbour.[1]

We shall have to go first to the Bible to see if this definition of health is adequate, and also to try and find there an answer to the problems raised in the last chapter.

God's plan for man

When we do so, the first pages of Genesis give us a very attractive picture. In God's creation, everything was good. He made loving provision of all that man could need, plants, fruit, animals and fish. Man and woman were together in a God-given unit.

They were told to be fruitful and fill the earth, but in doing so there would always be enough of everything they needed.

Central in their lives was their relationship to their Lord, giving them full freedom within the bounds of loving obedience.

Then came "lawlessness", to use St. John's word, and the whole pattern of life was shivered and fragmented. From now on every new endeavour would have a twist in it, each new society would carry in it the seeds of failure.

But God's people were given another chance to live in a manner that would be truly satisfying. The way of life that was sketched out for them by Moses has a special appeal today.

The Revised Scheme—a caring community

First of all, God was in the centre. Men were to love the Lord with all their hearts (*Deuteronomy* 6.5), and their happiness depended on whole-hearted obedience to him (*Deuteronomy* 28.1).

To obey meant victory, plenty and security, whereas disobedience would bring confusion, frustration and destruction. Everything depended on maintaining this close relationship of sons to a loving father.

Within this framework life was organized on a community basis. Every man was deeply conscious of the nation to which he belonged and also of his tribe, clan and family. His actions never affected himself alone. If he did what was right his children would benefit; if wrong, they would share in his punishment (*Numbers* 16.32). Such effects might still be felt ten generations later (*Deuteronomy* 23.2). He was part of a continuum stretching back through his forebears and forward to a long line of descendants and outwards into all the network of human relationships around him. Men differed in their tasks, their gifts of leadership and their skill, but all were part of the same fellowship and thus dependent on one another.

Compassion

It was a compassionate society, in spite of the undoubted harshness of some of its actions and punishments. Admittedly the people of the Canaanite cities were to be wholly destroyed (*Joshua* 6.21) and the "stubborn and rebellious son" or the adulterer faced the death penalty (*Deuteronomy* 21. 18–21). But these were strong measures to preserve Israel from "abominable practices", and from evils which would quickly spread.

In day-to-day life the Israelite was expected to be generous and caring towards his neighbour. When he reaped his fields he must not go to the very border; the gleanings were to be for the poor and the sojourner (*Leviticus* 19. 9–10). If he forgot a sheaf when reaping he should not go back; it was for the fatherless and the widow (*Deuteronomy* 24.19). Some of his olives and grapes must be left for others to take (*Deuteronomy* 24. 20–21).

Strangers who stayed with him deserved special consideration. The Jew knew the heart of a stranger, because of his experiences in Egypt, and so he must love the stranger as himself (*Exodus* 23.9).

In the same way he had a special responsibility for the fatherless and the widow, as the most vulnerable members of the family, and for the poor, the neediest group in the community. There must be no injustice to the fatherless, and the widow's garment must not be taken in pledge (*Deuteronomy* 24. 17).

If a poor man's cloak was taken as a surety for a loan, he must have it back at night to sleep in (*Deuteronomy* 24. 12). A poor Hebrew brother could not be made a slave, but must be treated as a hired servant, and that only for a limited period; in the year of jubilee he was to go back to his own family (*Leviticus* 25. 39–41).

The Jew was told to open his hand wide to the poor man and lend him whatever he needed, notwithstanding that he knew that every seven years all loans were to be cancelled. Ungrudging generosity would bring God's blessing (*Deuteronomy* 15. 7).

The same spirit of caring had to show itself in all sorts of practical ways. A man must build a parapet on his rooftop to prevent accidental falls (*Deuteronomy* 22.8), and if he found his neighbour's ox or sheep straying, he must return it (*Deuteronomy* 22. 1).

A life of moderation

Another leading characteristic of the God-directed life was moderation, or a spirit of conservation. The provision of the sabbath day, the sabbath year and the year of jubilee were examples of this.

The weekly day of rest was an interval of peace, freedom from stress and relaxation. And the seventh year was a "sabbath of solemn rest for the land", in which nothing was to be sown or reaped (*Leviticus* 25. 4). And every fiftieth year became another year of lying fallow (*Leviticus* 25. 11).

If the land was not allowed to rest in this way, it would claim its debt in the years to come, years in which it would be desolate, insisting on the repose which it had been denied before (*Leviticus* 26.33–35).

Living creatures deserved consideration too. The ox which was treading out the corn must be allowed to eat what he needed (*Deuteronomy* 25.4). If a bird's nest was found, the young could be taken but the mother must go free (*Deuteronomy* 22.6).

This moderation was especially valuable as regards the ownership of land and payment of debts. Every fifty years, in the year of jubilee, each man was restored to his property and his family. The land could not be sold in perpetuity, as it belonged to the Lord (*Leviticus* 25.13, 23).

And debts were cancelled every seven years. What a transformation it would bring if these laws could be applied in an Indian village or a township of North-East Brazil today!

In the same spirit of moderation a bridegroom was not drafted for military service for the first year of married life (*Deuteronomy* 24. 5). A Levite would "retire" at the age of fifty, it seems (*Numbers* 8.25). And the recurring feasts, the passover, the feasts of weeks and the feast of booths, each for a week or so at a time, meant regular family holidays with much enjoyment and hospitality (*Deuteronomy* 16).

All of this was to go on under the protection of God's blessing. There was no need to be anxious about food or rain or the future, as the Lord would take care of all these things (*Leviticus* 26. 3–13).

And social justice

A cornerstone of this balanced community living was social justice. Honesty was essential (*Exodus* 23.6). There was to be only one set of just weights and measures (*Deuteronomy* 25.15). Corrruption was forbidden and the poor man must be as fairly treated as the rich (*Exodus* 23. 6–8). The Israelites might make slaves of those of other nations and slavery was harsh, but these servants still had their rights. If a slave's tooth was knocked out by his master, the slave must be freed (*Exodus* 21.27). If a beautiful woman was taken as a slave but after a time was not wanted as a wife, she was free to go where she would (*Deuteronomy* 21.10–14).

In later years these principles were rejected and forgotten. Isaiah and Amos spoke bitterly of those who joined house to house and field to field till there was no more room: who trampled on the poor and turned aside the needy: who took bribes and falsified weights: and who bought slaves for the price of a pair of sandals. There was no justice then, no righteousness and no pity (*Isaiah* 5.7–8; *Amos* 5.11–12; 8.4–6).

Isaiah called the nation back to a fresh concern for those in need. If men would share their bread with the hungry, welcome the homeless poor and let the oppressed go free, life would be full of light and contentment and deep satisfaction (*Isaiah* 58.6–12).

Health as a result of right living

The teaching in the Old Testament on the marks of human society as it ought to be has been set out somewhat fully, because here health appears to be a by-product of right living, rather than a goal in itself.

A Godfearing community, compassionate in its relationships, caring for natural resources, setting its face against any divisions into rich and poor or between landowner and peasant, and holding firmly to principles of justice, is a community in which many of today's health problems would never arise.

Where health or healing are specifically mentioned (using the Hebrew word *rapha*) it is often in a figurative sense of restoring relationships or promoting peace (*Hosea* 14.4; *Isaiah* 57.18). The word *Shalom*, used once for healing, customarily describes peace and completeness, personal or national. A man rightly related to God and his fellows was normally a healthy man.

Of course there were sanitary laws governing "leprosy" (a different condition from the modern disease) and various discharges from the body. And rules about diet forbade the eating of swine (perhaps because of the risk of tape-worm cysts) and carrion birds like vultures or kites. This was all preventive medicine of a valuable kind.

But the physician was later on the scene and only appears in the Apocrypha (*Sirach* 38.1–15), and briefly elsewhere (2 *Chronicles* 16. 12).

It is true that the prophets performed miracles of healing. Elijah restored a widow's son to life (1 *Kings* 17. 17–24), and Elisha healed the Shunammite woman of barrenness, raised her son from the dead and cured Naaman of his leprosy (2 *Kings* 4 and 5).

These miracles, however, appear to be proofs of the God-given authority of the two prophets, possessed by them for a special purpose and time, and not to be repeated by others.

New Testament teaching

Healing was indeed prominent in the ministry of Jesus. He told the messengers of John the Baptist that as the result of his ministry the lame were walking, the lepers being cleansed and the deaf hearing (*St. Luke* 7.20–23). Wherever he went, sick people waited for him "in villages, cities or country" and many were made well (*St. Mark* 6.56). The blind saw, and the dead were raised (*St. John* 9.1–7; 11.43–44).

The disciples were given the same power to cure diseases (*St. Luke* 9.1–2 and 10.1, 8–9), and went preaching the gospel and healing everywhere (*St. Luke* 9. 6).

After the first Whit Sunday, the Apostles were able in the same way to heal the sick. Not only Peter and Paul did this, but Philip and Ananias too.

The power of Jesus as Saviour

What was the significance of this emphasis on healing? It surely was first a demonstration that Jesus had truly come as Saviour. When John the Baptist asks—"Are you the Christ, the one we are looking for?" Jesus answers—"Here is the proof: the lame walk, the deaf hear. . . ." How significant is one sentence in the story of the paralytic man. The scribes rejected Jesus' claim to forgive sins, and he replies "In order that you may know that the Son of man has authority on earth to forgive sins . . . rise (to the paralytic) and go home." The healing demonstrated that Jesus had the power to meet man's needs, however great (*St. Mark* 2.1–12).

At the same time his healings were instinctive acts of compassion for those whom he loved as whole people. Clearly he could not hesitate a moment before healing the man with the withered hand, or the woman bent double for 18 years. They had to be cured then and there in spite of the oppressive petty rules about the sabbath (*St. Luke* 6, 6–11; 13.10–17).

This love for men kept springing out in practical ways as Jesus went about "doing good and healing all that were oppressed by the devil", as Peter says (*Acts* 10.38).

The lives of the disciples

His followers were expected to have the same spirit. In the Sermon on the Mount, Jesus taught the importance of being meek and merciful, or as we would say today, showing unselfish kindness (*St. Matthew* 5.5–7).

The story of the Good Samaritan sums up unforgettably the way in which a man should obey the second commandment. Of course, he could and should show his compassion in other ways such as by feeding the hungry, for instance. But nothing depicts quite so much personal concern as touching and caring for a sick person (*St. Luke* 10.29–37).

Echoing the spirit of the Old Testament, the disciples of Jesus were taught to have a special caring for the poor (*St. Luke* 4.18), for children (*St. Mark* 9.37), and for rejected and despised groups (*St. Luke* 5.32). They were to be generous with their money (1 *Timothy* 6.18) and willing to share their possessions (*St. Luke* 6. 38).

It appears that Jesus and his early disciples performed miraculous acts of healing chiefly to demonstrate that they possessed a power of salvation which was equally able to redeem the souls or restore the bodies of their hearers.

By the time of the latter part of Acts, instances of miraculous healing appear to be rare, although Paul cured Publius with prayer and laying on of hands (*Acts* 28.8).

But Christians were still expected to have a healing ministry. Graham Swift considers that the great commission in *St. Mark* 16, which includes the ability to cure the sick by laying on of hands, is undoubtedly part of the teaching of scripture, even though the literary authenticity of the passage is uncertain.[3]

James laid it down that in sickness Christians should pray over the sick man and anoint him with oil, and the Lord would then raise him up (*James* 5. 14–15). And the ability to heal was one of the gifts of the Spirit (1 *Corinthians* 12.9).

But Paul was never cured of the "thorn in his flesh" (variously conjectured to be trachoma or recurrent attacks of malaria) in spite of much prayer (2 *Corinthians* 12.7–10). Timothy had "frequent ailments", for which Paul prescribed a little wine! (1 *Timothy* 5.23). And Luke the beloved physician had his place at Paul's side (*Colossians* 4.14).

Perhaps the lesson is that Christians should pray earnestly about sickness just as about other matters; that sometimes such prayer and laying on of hands, either by a group of mature Christians or by those to whom the Holy Spirit gives special ability, will effect a complete cure, and that even if this does not happen, such prayer will bring great benefits.

But it appears that at the same time men were expected to use ordinary means of treatment and care. And sometimes God would allow the sickness to continue as part of his plan—a plan that we cannot fully understand, though we see pointers to it.

Death itself was not a disaster but a gateway to glory, the way to become a "man of heaven", the last step before inheriting the Kingdom of God (1 *Corinthians* 15. 43, 48,50).

The attitude of Jesus and his disciples to health is a paradoxical one. They responded to sickness and suffering with compassion and love, in contrast to the cold indifference of the Pharisees. But for themselves they met suffering and even death willingly, sometimes joyfully. As in the Old Testament, obedience to God and a loving relationship with him counted for more than physical health. But a concern for healing—a responsibility for the health of a brother or sister—that was another matter, and an obligation that could not be shirked.

A loving community

The New Testament is like the Old in emphasizing "man in community". We are part of a great living fellowship of which Christ is the glorious Head, and in which we all have our distinct but interlocking roles. This God-given community, the Church, must act in a special way if it is to be true to itself.

Its members must have the mind of Christ, unselfish, loving, humble and self-sacrificing (*Philippians* 2.1–11). They must "wash one another's feet", loving and serving one another in any humble way that offers itself, as Jesus commanded (*St. John* 13.14–15). And they must attest the reality of their discipleship by generous sharing of their possessions with those in need (1 *John* 3.17–18.

James 2.15–17). Such deeds are the essential evidence that proves whether a man is a genuine Christian or not.

Jesus' picture of the Great Judgment tells the same story. The faith of men is tested by Him, not on the grounds of what they say, but through the record of their acts of practical love for those in want.

In this great drama the practice of "healing" broadens out into any kind of care which an ordinary man could give to a neighbour in trouble. And such care is the touchstone which demonstrates whether a man's faith rings true or whether it is just a sham (*St. Matthew* 25.31–46).

To sum up, both in the Old and New Testaments the people of God form a special society, compassionate to the poor and weak, sensitive to each other's needs, unselfish and generous.

In the New Testament this loving attitude turns outwards from the Church to the community around, giving the same practical help to the stranger as to the brother in Christ. And this is not something for the few who have a special interest in it, but is the indispensable hallmark of a true Christian faith.

References **Chapter 2**

1. de Pury, Pascal. op cit.
2. MacNutt, Francis. *Healing*, Ave Maria Press, Notre Dame, Indiana, 1974. p. 56.
3. Swift, C. E. Graham, *The New Bible Commentary Revised.* Inter-Varsity Press, London, 1970. p. 886.

Chapter 3

DREAMING DREAMS

"If there were dreams to sell,
Merry and sad to tell,
What would you buy?" *Dream Pedlary*, T. L. Beddoes.

"What would I do if I could begin all over again?" wrote Merfyn Temple, looking back on 30 years work as a Methodist missionary with a special interest in rural development.[1]

"I would question my Western-culture-based assumptions", he affirms; "I would spend far more time listening to, and trying to understand, the contemporary wisdom of rural people . . . I would read much more carefully what Jesus said about the conditions of blessedness . . . I would dream more about the New Jerusalem and share my dreams . . . I would trust the local congregation more, asking it to worship and pray more: I would lead them into the field to dig conservation works and spread muck on the land."

What have other men been dreaming nowadays about the way in which Christians should care for their fellow men?

Cosmic planning

Robert Lambourne and James Mathers, Christian psychiatrists who worked for many years in Birmingham, have the gift of stimulating others to think, and I shall quote extensively from them.

We should have a wide perspective, insists Mathers,[2] and work on a broad canvas.

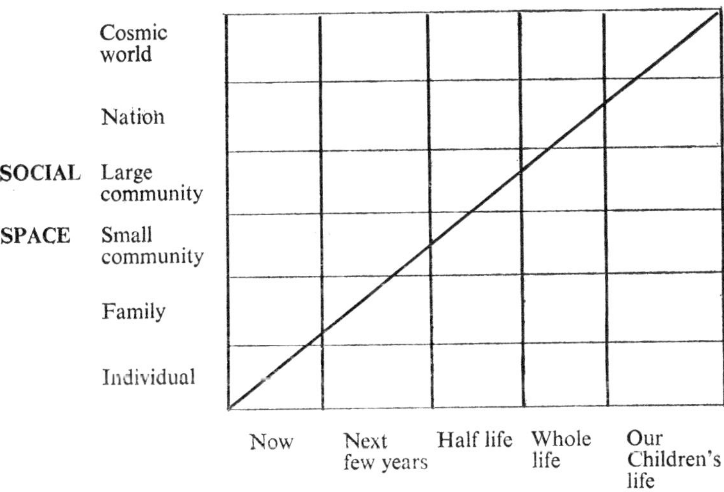

He illustrates his thesis by the above diagram. We may be limited in our work to a fairly small area, he explains, but in perspectives we should move over a wide field. It is easier to concentrate on the bottom left-hand corner but we should be planning a strategy which reaches far up and to the right.

He spells this strategy out for the doctor and nurse in a second and similar diagram, modified from a chart of Lambourne's.

SOCIAL SPACE						
(World) Nation						Theologian or Visionary
Large community					Health Adviser	
Small community		Community Psychiatrist		Therapeutic Community		
Family		Paediatrician			G.P.	
Whole person		Physician	Nurse			
Organ of body or cell	Surgeon Micro-biologist					
	Eradicating disease	Managing disease	Caring for sufferer	Learning by suffering	Nurturing existing strengths	Creating new style of being

INCREASING DEGREE OF PERSONAL INVOLVEMENT

Much medical work, asserts Mathers, is concentrated again in the lower left-hand corner. The microbiologist finds the organism which causes the disease, or the surgeon removes the diseased appendix. These are the "doers".

But many illnesses are chronic or recurrent; and these have to be "managed", cared for over a long period before they respond to treatment. For the old or the mentally handicapped there may be no complete cure, and it is care rather than cure that is needed, the special responsibility of the nurse.

In the therapeutic community of a psychiatric hospital, the members learn the lessons of their illnesses from one another. A good general practitioner, like a good teacher, will bring out a patient's latent ego strength and build it up, to cope with the stresses and limitations of illness. And the visionary, theological or medical, plans a style of living which is truly human.

The "doers" are more greatly esteemed than the "planners", but we should all be planners, balanced and adaptable, giving all concepts of treatment their rightful place.

Joys of living

Shortly before his death in 1972, Bob Lambourne wrote again on the philosophy of medical care, with particular emphasis on his own specialty of psychiatry.[3]

He began by tracing the way in which the teachings of public health and preventive medicine had steadily grown in importance in medical thinking.

Forty years or so ago public health was a distinct but limited discipline, just one subject in the medical curriculum. Gradually it gained in importance, as first the paediatrician and the obstetrician, and then the physician and the surgeon realized more and more the importance of the prevention of disease.

Stage by stage, typhoid fever, tuberculous joints and the deformities of poliomyelitis disappeared from the hospital wards. Today public health plays an essential part in all specialties. As a result it gives to health a "political" aspect, and interacts with agriculture, education and industry, each new development in one producing a change in all the rest.

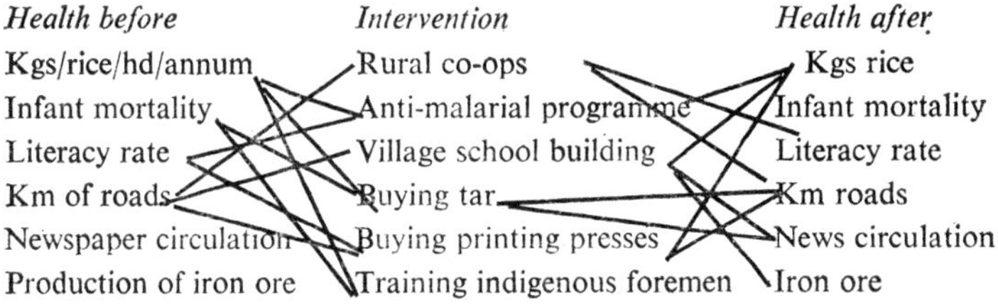

Now the emphasis has been switched from the individual to the community. Health and justice cannot be separated. Health then becomes built into the fabric of daily living, as the following diagram demonstrates.

<table>
<tr><td colspan="2">Surgery</td><td rowspan="3">H
o
u
s
i
n
g</td><td colspan="2">Education</td></tr>
<tr><td colspan="2">Industry</td><td colspan="2">Entertainment</td></tr>
<tr><td colspan="2">Communications</td><td colspan="2">Paediatrics</td></tr>
<tr><td>Mid-
wifery</td><td colspan="2">Law and
Order</td><td>Agri-
culture</td><td>Defence</td></tr>
</table>

But, says Lambourne, health in this scheme declares itself as a political matter, a material possession to which every man has a right.

To this materialistic view of health, psychiatry introduces a new dimension. It too began as a limited relatively minor specialty in the medical student's curriculum. Little by little the importance of psychiatry in the management of a variety of diseases became appreciated, until now psychiatric concepts are changing the whole attitudes of psychiatrists to health.

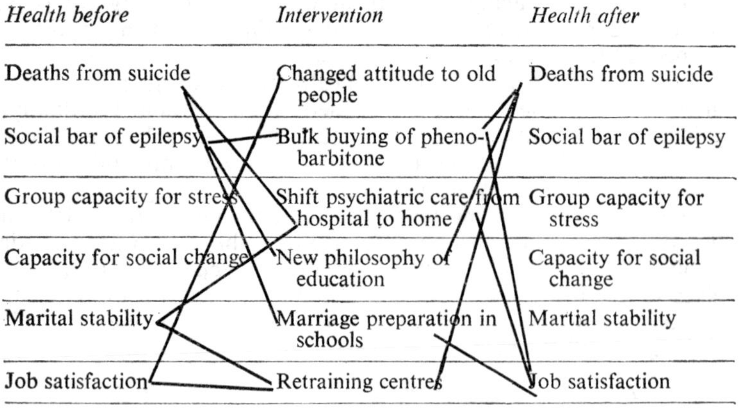

Health before	*Intervention*	*Health after*
Deaths from suicide	Changed attitude to old people	Deaths from suicide
Social bar of epilepsy	Bulk buying of phenobarbitone	Social bar of epilepsy
Group capacity for stress	Shift psychiatric care from hospital to home	Group capacity for stress
Capacity for social change	New philosophy of education	Capacity for social change
Marital stability	Marriage preparation in schools	Martial stability
Job satisfaction	Retraining centres	Job satisfaction

Again each form of intervention interacts with each health situation, to produce widespread changes for the better.

The style of life which results, says Lambourne, is obedient, imaginative and humble: health is "a surprising joy to which every human being comes by grace."

He now sees health as "an ideal state of souls in fellowship", part of a pattern of living in which "health" and "wholeness" cannot be separated from one another.

<table>
<tr><td>Surgery</td><td rowspan="2">Family</td><td colspan="2">Learning</td></tr>
<tr><td rowspan="2">Sacrifice</td><td colspan="2">Joy</td></tr>
<tr><td></td><td colspan="2">Mercy</td></tr>
<tr><td colspan="2">Communication</td><td colspan="2">Anger</td></tr>
<tr><td rowspan="2">Midwifery</td><td rowspan="2">Agape</td><td>Wonder</td><td>Art</td></tr>
<tr><td>Respon-sibility</td><td>Community</td><td>Dance</td></tr>
</table>

Health is now combined with other joys of living to form a community in a state of well-being.

Pressing his argument home to medical missionaries, Lambourne recalls that very little has been done in missionary enterprise to promote mental health.

We must balance, says he, the undoubted benefits of comprehensive health care, where the emphasis is often on inexpensive treatment and wide effectiveness, with a deep concern for people as persons, not forgetting the patient with mental handicap say, who can contribute little in economic terms, but whom the community certainly needs.

Dreaming dreams, planning for long periods of time ahead, caring as well as curing, strengthening individual resources, aiming to make a community both healthy and loving—these are some of the emphases we have studied so far.

For Jesus' sake

What other principles are there to guide us in forming a picture of what Christian health care should be?

First, because it is Christian care, Jesus must be acknowledged as Lord. Only He can give real life and complete the picture of full well-being. In the Kingdom of Heaven He is King. The nation's health service will of course be secular and Christians will co-operate fully with it. But the work done by the Christian Church will be for Jesus' sake.

Man's dignity

Then each man will be viewed as a person whose dignity must be respected. President Nyerere stresses this in the Arusha Declaration[4] and President Kaunda has said the same. If a man is poor and a peasant, then he has the greater claim for respect. He should be served with consideration and consulted and listened to. James Mathers affirms that everyone has an equal right to be heard in a matter of health, whoever he is. And the voice of those for whom the system is *not* working, such as peasants or the mentally ill, should be listened to most earnestly of all.[5]

In family-planning campaigns, for instance, as Bishop Sadiq has said, decisions must not be made on socio-economic grounds alone, with the inducement of payment for the right results.[6] Couples should be invited to make up their minds as responsible parents and urged to show altruism and consideration for others, not least for the welfare of their children to be. And my neighbour, my patient must be seen as a whole being, not only as someone who is physically ill, nor again only as a soul. In Hebrew thought man was a unity, a complete person, and this is the picture of the New Testament too. African beliefs are just the same. The physical, mental and spiritual characteristics of a man are interwoven and cannot be fully separated.

Man's self-reliance is to be fostered, so that the success of any scheme should be judged by the extent to which it builds up local initiative. Even in sickness, the patient should act in a fully responsible way.

Persons in Community

After the individual comes the community. Indeed the Old Testament, as Lambourne says, swings between the community and the person and any complete separation of the two is a false one.

The relationships of mother and child, or husband and wife, produce illness in each other. A patient brings with him a whole series of relationships which affect his illness and his symptoms. In treatment he needs the support of the group to which he belongs. He cannot be seen in isolation from other people, all people.

Here the traditional strength of the family and clan in Africa provides the succour which he needs.

The Western-trained doctor or nurse cannot see any place for the patient's relative within the work of the ward. It is the nurses who should care for the patient, feed him and make him comfortable.

But the patient and his wife or sister know that, special diets apart, the food tastes better if she has cooked it, that no one can give the little attentions as well and as often as she can, and that the familiar face and voice, the news from home, and the reassurance that all is going well there in his absence are powerful aids in helping him towards recovery.

The West is gradually learning what Africa at least has always known, that the family can be the greatest of strengths in illness.

Rejection and loneliness

But yet this is not always so. Perhaps family quarrels have been part of the trouble. Or the disease is of a kind such as leprosy or mental illness, which the relatives greatly fear.

Here the Christian community should play its part, and give the support and friendship which the patient needs.

This is not easy, as Joyce Peel of Madras tells us.[7]

"Visiting the TB hospital," she writes, "is my main personal contact with pain and suffering. It is not just the disease, which is terrible enough, but the effect it has on the family. Many of these women have been deserted by their husbands, who take other wives or women who do not care for the first wife's children. If there is no remarriage, then even so the children are neglected. Many patients are unvisited, and get no letters, and nothing is given them to do. They sit on their beds and worry, and this worry wears them out and hurries on their disease.

"If only I could help them turn their worry into prayer. My utter helplessness throws me back on God and I can only cry 'Here I am, Lord; please communicate something of your love for them through me.'

"Just now the power cut means the fans don't work and so the patients are irritated by mosquitoes. The pastor and I are wondering what we can do. There doesn't seem much. I wish we could find someone to teach the patients some activity. I gave them ludo to play and they play it every night."

Perhaps it will usually be individual Christians who care deeply in this way. But whole groups can learn such practical loving, as is described later in this book.

And most of all, Christians could help the dying patient to meet death without fear. As Christians we should encounter death with an active acceptance of God's will, an affirmation that death is the most important moment in life, that there can indeed be hope and peace and a New Creation waiting.

But we are so frail, so easily afraid, and the last journey can be so lonely. We so greatly need the support of friends and brothers as we enter our last life-situation and make our "last thrust to the Father". We want the strength of human nearness, a voice and the grasp of a warm hand, the comfort of knowing that we shall not be left alone.

This is the spirit of Mother Teresa who says of those who are dying on the streets of Calcutta, "we want them to know that there are people who really love them, who really want them . . . that they are the children of God and that they are loved and cared about.

"What we are doing is just a drop in the ocean. But if that drop was not in the ocean, I think the ocean will be less because of that missing drop. It was worth while having that home (for the dying) even for those few people to die beautifully, with God and in peace."[8]

References **Chapter 3**

1. Temple, Merfyn. *Rural Development Bulletin*, June 15 1974, CMS, London.
2. Mathers, James. *Strategy and Tactics of Health Care: Reflections on the 'Concepts Map'* (awaiting publication).
3. Lambourne, Robert. "Mental Health, Christian Medical Mission and Comprehensive Health Care", *Religion and Medicine*, **2**, SCM, London, 1973.
4. Nyerere, Julius. *Arusha Declaration.*
5. Mathers, James. op cit.
6. Sadiq, Bishop J. W. *Contact* 22 Christian Family Planning, CMC, Geneva, 1974.
7. Peel, Joyce. Link Letter, March 1973, CMS, London.
8. Muggeridge, Malcolm. *Something Beautiful for God*, Fontana, London, 1972.

Chapter 4

HAPPY FAMILIES

"*All happy families resemble each other.*" Tolstoy

The importance of the family for health and happiness, says Dr. Halfdan Mahler, Director-General of the World Health Organization, is hard to exaggerate. The early years of life from pregnancy onwards are so very important.

It is the family that more than anything else determines a child's chance of realizing his full talents, Dr Mahler continues. At home a child learns all the time without realizing it, through his relationships with his parents and grandparents, through the talk that goes on around him, and through all the ways in which he is encouraged to be self-reliant.[1]

So the family should be the first target for health care. But before attempting to give such care, doctors and nurses must listen and learn. They must study the life-style of the community, understand what is currently believed about health and disease, and discover what home treatments are given for everyday illnesses.[2]

We must find out, urges Una Maclean, doctor and anthropologist, about food habits, preferred family size, and the culture in general of our families, if effective medical care is to be given at household level.[3]

From such studies will come comprehension of the felt needs which parents have, and of ways in which these needs can best be met. And then we can go on to win the confidence and support of the mothers in the community.

Mothers first

A writer in the *New Internationalist* reflecting on Women's Year, 1975, emphasizes that it is women who grow most of the food in the Third World, especially in Africa. Population studies, too, shew that the birthrate in any country is closely related to the position of women in that community.

And rural development, rural employment, the level of public health, and the standard of child care, all depend for successful progress on a change in the present unjust position of women in society. A full recognition of women's role is essential to world development.[4]

So the mother must be central in any programme of health care. And without question, every mother wants to do the best for her child. On her breast milk he thrives. When he is weaned, it is she who will grow most of his food, she who will cook it, she who will care lovingly for him and treat his childhood illnesses. Maybe she needs to learn improved ways of providing such care. But love is a great teacher, and her motives to do better are strong.

Fathers must not be left out however. In most traditional societies it is the man who makes decisions about what food should be eaten, and the number of children his wife will have, at the same time being guided himself by the traditions of the clan and the tribe. Fathers must be consulted about new ideas on better nutrition or methods of family spacing.

The Beautiful Flower

Two nutrition projects in Africa illustrate the importance of this "family" approach. The first is Mwanamugimu, the Malnutrition Rehabilitation Centre in Kampala, Uganda. The name is borrowed from a Luganda proverb "The beautiful flower comes from healthy roots." Two doctors in particular, Paget Stanfield and Michael Church, planned this clinic in the army hut-like buildings of the old Mulago Hospital on the outskirts of the city, buildings that stood empty when patients moved across into the handsome new six-storey block close by.[5]

Stanfield and Church were distressed by the number of toddlers in central Uganda who suffered and died from protein-calorie malnutrition, often known as kwashiorkor. The problem, as they saw it, was one of education. If mothers could be convinced that their children were not suffering from a mysterious illness needing injections and medicine, but merely required different food, they would quickly cure their own babies and teach the method to others. So the old wards were turned into dormitories and demonstration rooms, and mothers were invited to bring their malnourished children for a three-week stay. As far as possible women were chosen who were influential in their communities, and who came from areas where malnutrition was common.

The new arrivals found mothers like themselves demonstrating the cooking of children's meals—not very different from their ordinary diet, but with beans or sweet bananas added. The kitchen was just like the one they used at home. Firewood was burning in the stove, the saucepans were the familiar type, and when quantities of food were talked about, no complicated measures were given but just "a handful" of maize flour or "a big spoonful" of beans.

During the day there were talks on child feeding by the staff, visits to the nearby market, and of course their own meals and their babies' meals to prepare. They saw their children improve daily on nothing more than the new mixed diet. Soon they were taking their turn in demonstrating and explaining correct feeding to the next batch of newcomers.

While they were learning all this at Mwanamugimu, their homes were visited by members of staff who spoke to the fathers, and then met with local chiefs and religious leaders to explain what the women might be expected to do on their return. Each mother on leaving the Centre was encouraged to be an active nutrition educator in her community, organizing a women's club for this purpose if she possibly could, and of course cooking the new mixed meals in her own home. A member of staff would call on her from time to time, to see how much she had been able to influence her neighbours.

Jane Neville, a missionary occupational therapist who visited Mwanamugimu, learnt from the doctor in charge how its success had been achieved.[6]

Firstly, the staff had carried out a detailed study of the customs and beliefs of the people concerned in matters of health, food, disease and pregnancy. Then the work done was in response to a felt need of the community. Everyone had seen children who were ill with kwashiorkor, and knew that some of them had died. Again ordinary people were themselves involved in the programme. Each mother went home with her healthy child, ready with her answer when her neighbour asked a wondering "How?"—ready to teach the secret that would keep other children fit and well fed.

And lastly the personality of the workers ensured success—all were actively interested in the project and full of enthusiasm.

School for Parents

A similar family-based movement was begun in NW Rwanda some years ago by Suzanne Chiasson, a dynamic French-Canadian nurse.[7] Again the problem was kwashiorkor, malnutrition from lack of protein and calories in the recently-weaned child.

Suzanne made the parents take an active part in the treatment—something they had never done before. The mothers were told to bring their babies every month—a different day of the month being allotted to each of the surrounding hilltop communities. On arrival there would be a talk on the right kind of food for toddlers, then a free discussion, followed by a look at the demonstration food garden and the chickens and rabbits. Each baby was weighed and the weight plotted on a chart which the mother kept.

On another visit the mother would cook a sample meal. Remarkably, this school for parents insisted on a two year course, with an examination at the end, taken very seriously. Fathers had to join the school too, and would learn the way to build a latrine.

During the course the attitude of the mothers would change. They knew now that kwashiorkor was not due to poisoning. They became confident that they could feed their children properly, and would teach other mothers the way to do it. Sister Suzanne noted that subsequent children born in these families were well-fed and free from kwashiorkor. And the young girls whom she trained as "monitrices" (instructors) taught the same lessons throughout northern Rwanda.

"We must win the families, including the extended families", say Drs. Rex and Jeanne Blumhagen: "we should concentrate on them more than on individuals, strengthening the solidarity of each family and fostering self-reliance."[8]

References — Chapter 4

1. Mahler, Halfdan, Address to the National Council of International Health, Washington, October 16 1974.
2. Matthews, C. M. E. *Journal of the Christian Medical Association of India*, 1974, **49,** p. 328.
3. Maclean, Una, Report of Applied Technological Conference, University of Edinburgh, September 1973 (mimeo).
4. *New Internationalist*, April 1975, p. 26.
5. Stanfield, J. Paget, ed. "Recent Approaches to Malnutrition in Uganda", Monograph 13, reprint from *The Journal of Tropical Pediatrics and Environmental Child Health*, 1971, **17,** pp. 1–88.
6. Neville, Jane. Report of Health Education Tour, May–June 1971. ALERT PO Box 165, Addis Ababa.
7. Chiasson, Suzanne. *Journal Medical au Rwanda*, Janvier 1971.
8. Blumhagen, Rex and Jeanne. *Medical Missions' Role in Health Care Delivery.* Refer to Medical Assistance Programs Inc., Wheaton, Ill. (mimeo).

Chapter 5

WIDENING THE CIRCLE

It is only a small step from the family to the community and here doctors have to beware. "Community medicine", wrote William Foege, himself a physician, "is far too important to be entrusted to the medical profession. In general one good agriculturalist is better than ten physicians in a developing country. And sanitary (public health) engineers are more valuable than doctors . . . in the same surroundings."[1]

This is not the kind of thing that medical people like to hear. But if by "doctors" Foege means those who do almost entirely curative work, it is hard to resist his logic.

The health of a community depends largely on a moderate degree of prosperity, together with good farming methods, opportunities for work, and the informed good sense of the whole population, as well as on cleanliness, pure water and other health measures.

Jesus has a "both/and"

Christian Rural Service in East Africa has valuable lessons to teach about this balanced development of all sides of everyday life.

Dick Lyth, one time soldier and District Commissioner in the Sudan and later missionary leader and bishop, was troubled in the early 1960s by the situation in Kigezi in SW Uganda, the country where he was working.[2]

Nearly half the population was under the age of sixteen, illiteracy rates were high, (up to 80% in women), poverty was oppressive, and disease was widespread.

Jesus had a both/and in his contact with people, Dick reflected. "Your sins are forgiven", said Jesus and then "rise up and walk." So religion and compassion must go together.

But he saw big gaps in this compassion. The church had provided pastoral care, schools, even hospitals. But what about farming, nutrition and improvement in the standard of living?

Shouldn't church members be able to improve their health, their homes and their farms?

So with the help of World Neighbours and Christian Aid, two very imaginative donor agencies, a new scheme was launched. Young men with better than average education and an infectious Christian faith were trained briefly in a variety of skills and sent off two by two, each with a bicycle, camp bed and cooking pot, to work in key parishes.

The first step was to teach adults to write. Then came protected springs. In each place where water bubbled out from a spring, a small dam was needed, with an outlet pipe and a roofing layer of stones and earth, to protect the water from being fouled. The

Government were willing to give cement and the pipe if neighbouring people would collect sand and stones, and ten Ugandan shillings (50p, $1.00) to pay the mason.

The scheme had lagged until Christian Rural Service workers came along and enthused everybody, working with them and providing the know-how.

Then came Sunday schools, bicycle repairs, advice on keeping rabbits and chickens, and soil conservation.

Smallholders were encouraged to work together and pool money to buy pesticides or form a credit and loan society.

Health work included teaching the basics of hygiene, nutrition, first aid and family planning. The workers co-operated with the Government medical service, and supported the smallpox vaccination campaigns.

Help was given in building latrines and Dick called his men the privy counsellors! Encouraging village industries, stocking fish ponds, starting Young Farmers' Clubs, and preaching the Gospel whenever there was an opportunity—this was the way the Service grew.

The ultimate aim, said Dick, was that this practical concern for others, showing them "the kindness of God", as King David had said, should become part of the everyday life of the Church, carried out largely by volunteers.

Planning in Bhagyanagar

This same concern for all sides of life has been demonstrated by Andrew Bulmer, working at close range in Bhagyanagar village in Orissa, eastern India.[3] There are 200 people in the village, 30 being Brahmins and fairly well off, while the remaining 170 are Harijan ('Children of the Gods': former outcastes) who earn about 20p ($0.40) a day and own no land.

Andrew, aged 26 and working for the Volunteer Relief Organization, VRO, has been planning what he ought to do. He knows that a volunteer worker cannot dominate, but must aim for "interdependence", his ideas and vision being matched by the villagers' practical knowledge. So how should he begin?

His first goals were to learn the language, know every villager and child by name and know all about their circumstances. Then he recalled that VRO's original aim had been to rebuild houses in villages like this one which had been badly damaged by hurricanes. So strongly built houses are first on his list.

Next he wanted a baseline survey. He planned a "Family Album", with a family photo on each page and below it information about the household. Other smaller surveys would deal with employment, health and education and give maps of plots and trees.

What about finance? It was essential to build up a community fund, so as to give a reserve for any new venture or unforeseen crisis.

Better conditions of employment were very important too. To improve their farming prospects, the landless labourers ought to join a co-operative, so as to cultivate land owned by the community. Poultry farming, fish ponds, spinning and weaving were other valuable ways to earn a living.

And then came health. A survey would include the examination of each person, a health diagnosis for the whole community, a nutrition survey and plans for health education.

The remaining goals were effective education, an active village council, and time for books, music and drama.

Health was thus set in the broad framework of the whole life and advancement of the village. And the keys to success were self-sufficiency or self-reliance, and "togetherness".

In successive articles in *The New Internationalist* Andrew has vividly described the difficulties and delays that he met in putting his ideas into practice.

Making life richer

There seems no doubt that health care at family and community level is one among many ways in which life is made fuller and richer—an important way indeed, but not to be carried on in isolation.

Reuel Stallones speaks of a "synthetic" approach to health. In the past, he says, disease and mortality were reduced through a general improvement in the quality of life, brought about in various ways without any particular planning. And in future many different influences will work together in the same way so that better health results.[4]

So it is and will be in SW Uganda and Bhagyanagar, with better housing, better jobs and better education all playing their important parts in making life freer from preventable disease.

Health care in China in the last 25 years teaches the same lesson. The mass health campaigns that have had such impressive results were never undertaken in isolation. They were always linked with other mass campaigns, in agriculture, for instance.

In the Chinese commune, comprising an average of 10,000 people, afforestation and the building of dams and reservoirs, or the making of simple farm tools and supplies of fertiliser, rank in importance side by side with the eradication of smallpox, the campaign against rats and mosquitoes and the elimination of bilharzia, as is more fully explained in Chapter 7.

Joint Christian groups working in developing countries have adopted the same broad approach. ACROSS (Africa Committee for Rehabilitation of the Southern Sudan), a consortium of several missionary societies to provide much needed help at the end of the long civil war in that country, has a medical programme of out-patient clinics, mobile units and hospital work. But it wants its nurses to join the community development teams which aim to "educate for living", by helping in building houses, teaching better cooking and improving water supplies. Training young people for jobs as blacksmiths, tailors or dressmakers, carpenters and motor mechanics is all part of the programme.[5]

And HEED (Health, Education and Economic Development) in Bangladesh, another joint venture by missionary societies and relief agencies, is as interested in housing, jute growers' co-operatives, and handicrafts as it is in providing health care.[6]

Let the community make the plans

All such schemes, however, depend for their success on long and painstaking discussion with community leaders until the new ideas are gradually accepted and a change of behaviour takes place.

The Indian Government has carried out a massive well-drilling programme during the last ten years. But many of the wells are reported not to be working, because a new technology was imposed on a deep rooted and traditional society, without enough effort being made to consult the village and explain exactly what was going to be done.[7]

Christine Matthews, formerly research physicist and now missionary health educator at Vellore, South India, urges that changing the behaviour of people is difficult and certain principles must never be forgotten.

"Work through leaders and group influences", she stresses. "The social influence of others in the group is very important.

"Ensure the participation of the community", she continues, "right from the planning stage. Let the community decide the priorities and how much help they need. And meet felt needs first."[8]

These lessons from her experience, hammered out by living for two years in a small South Indian village, are widely endorsed by many planners today.

The immensely important art of helping any community of people to achieve a higher standard of health and happiness calls for great resources of humility, patience and understanding.

References **Chapter 5**

1. Foege, William, *Community Medicine*. CMC/70/17, Christian Medical Commission, Geneva.
2. Lyth, R. *Mission to the Under-loved,* Ruanda CMS, London.
3. Bulmer, Andrew. *New Internationalist,* November 1974 and January, February, March 1975; and circular letter of 19.7.74.
4. Stallones, Reuel. *Science*, 1972, **175,** No. 4021.
5. ACROSS programme dated July 1974. Nairobi and Juba.
6. HEED paper by Tear Fund (mimeo) 14.11.74, Teddington, Middlesex.
7. "Water", *New Internationalist*, February 1975.
8. Matthews, C. M. E. *Journal of Christian Medical Association of India*, 1974, **49,** p. 328.

Chapter 6

TAKING HEALTH TO WHERE IT IS NEEDED MOST

Close to the country palace of the late King "Freddy" of Buganda, (whose proper title was Kabaka Edward Mutesa II) is Luteete Maternity and Child Health Centre. It is in gently-rolling cotton- and coffee-growing country, 30 miles from Kampala, the capital of Uganda.

Lessons from Luteete

Here for many years Mengo Hospital, belonging to the Anglican Church of Uganda, has had a health outpost. In recent times Drs. Paget Stanfield, one time professor of child health at Makerere University, and Michael Church developed it into a model community health centre with many striking features.[1]

They agreed with Dr. Fred Sai of Ghana that the five health priorities for Africa were—

Good antenatal care for all pregnant mothers
Proper nutrition of children under 5
Immunization of small children against the common infectious diseases
General health education, especially of parents
and Family Planning advice

The centre of Luteete's work therefore was the "Under-Fives Clinic" for small children aged under five years, or rather the Family Clinic as it should be called, because mothers were very much included.

Such clinics were held regularly near the older-established small ward and dispensary unit, using a separate clinic building, the cement blocks of which had been paid for by the local Men's Club.

This building had low half-walls, a sensible saving in cost in a hot country. Mothers sat on low plank seats, so that with babies on their laps their feet were comfortably on the ground.

Each mother brought her baby's weight-chart, the well-known "Road to Health" of David Morley, which shows the broad-banded graph of satisfactory weight-gain in the first years of life, and on this the baby's own weight was plotted at each visit. Between visits the mother kept the card in a plastic wallet.

BCG immunization against tuberculosis, smallpox vaccination, polio vaccine given by mouth, triple vaccine to protect against diphtheria, whooping cough and tetanus, and measles vaccine when this expensive injection could be afforded, were all recorded on the chart with dates.

Daily group talks and individual teaching were given, stressing correct feeding and general hygiene. Standard treatment was provided for the common illnesses of childhood, it being accepted that prevention and treatment could not be separated in such a clinic. Tablets were pre-packed to save time in dispensing, and simple fluid medicines were ladled out into the mother's waiting bottle, using a ladle of known capacity.

As it was a family clinic, pregnant women were examined and advised, and any who were "at risk" because of small stature, contracted pelvis, history of a previous difficult labour and so on were specially "starred" for delivery under skilled supervision. At a post-natal visit mothers were given family planning advice.

A small laboratory had been set up where routine haemoglobin tests for anaemia and stool tests for parasites were carried out.

Mother and child progressed through the clinic step by step, from reception clerk to nurse, then perhaps to the doctor or to ante-natal examination room, laboratory, injection room, and dispensary.

Around and behind the clinic building were first model latrines, one being child's size with a small opening in the concrete plinth, so that a child could learn to use a latrine without the real danger of a fall through a large opening into the pit below.

From time to time a big bore-hole auger was demonstrated, by which a man could cut an adequate hole for a latrine pit in a few hours, instead of having all the labour of a conventionally-dug pit. Of course the auger would have to be co-operatively owned.

Next, the kitchens were of the model raised kind. When food is cooked in a pot balanced on three stones with the fire in the centre, as is the popular way, a toddler can trip and fall on the pot and fire, and many are admitted to hospital with severe scalds and burns. A raised cooking surface had been built of bricks, and was fired by sticks fed into the hollow centre of the stove from the side; this proved itself to be safe for children and more efficient for the mother. Here mothers would cook demonstration protein meals for children, to be sampled in the clinic.

Close by stood a nutritional rehabilitation unit, a simple house built very cheaply with rammed earth bricks made from the plentiful "murram" or ironstone earth around, mixed with a small proportion —say 5%—of cement, and compressed hard in a Cinva ram. Here mothers would stay if their babies were suffering from severe malnutrition, so as to be under the nurses' eyes. It was not, however, used as much as had been hoped.

Beside it were chicken coops and rabbit hutches, easy to make, and very effective. A little further on stood the cattle kraal, set up by university staff to study whether a young farmer could feed one or two cows on the elephant grass around, cutting it daily; if he were successful it would prove that a smallholder could make a living from selling the milk and still have enough for his family besides.

Further back lay the demonstration food plots, carefully contoured and with adequate irrigation channels, all prepared by Luke, the experienced cultivator and health educator. Parents attending the clinics were encouraged to find out how they could grow protein-rich vegetables for themselves.

Half a mile away in the valley was a protected spring. This had been built by the initiative of the Men's Club associated with the Health Centre, a club chaired by the vicar and meeting regularly to discuss new community ventures. The triumph of the spring lay in the fact that the whole local community, Protestant, Catholic and Muslim, had joined in making it, with the chief himself putting on his shorts so as to carry stones more energetically.

It was a great day when everyone gathered with beaming smiles to see their work completed, and clean water flowing out of the pipe just at the right height for a waiting kerosene tin or calabash.

Home visiting was another feature of the Health Centre. From it the Assistant Health Visitor would visit homes of patients who lived within walking distance, to see if the parents were keeping up the child's immunizations and giving him the right food. She would enquire tactfully whether they had tried making a safe kitchen, and if the latrine was being regularly used.

I have described Luteete in detail because of the many impressive innovations which it brought out,—new ideas which attracted visitors from long distances.

It was intended to be fully reproducible and this was true of its individual activities. But the Centre as a whole, with its links with the University, inevitably had a research and teaching aspect which meant that highly-skilled visiting staff gave much time to it, transport costs were substantial, and ventures like the cattle kraal had to be subsidized. It was, in short, bigger and more expensive than an ordinary rural community could afford.

Also, it had not been able to achieve a satisfactory relationship with the Government community development centre across the road, though much would have been gained if the two units had joined forces. Luteete nevertheless has been a powerful stimulus to practical effort in comprehensive community health.

Community health at Ludhiana

In North India, at Ludhiana Christian Medical College, the approach to better community health began differently.[2] Leaders in the College reflected on John Bryant's words—"half the world has no health care: and for many, the health care received doesn't meet their need."[3] And also on David Morley's rule of "three-quarters"—"three-quarters of the population of developing countries live in rural areas, but three-quarters of the medical resources are in the towns, where three-quarters of the doctors live: three-quarters of the deaths are from preventable disease, but three-quarters of medical budgets are spent on curative medicine."[4]

This rule holds true for India where 80% of the population live in the villages.

How were the difficulties of India to be overcome—the conservatism of the villager, the fatalism that accepted subnormal health as natural, the presence of several varieties of traditional medical philosophy, such as Unani and Vedic, and the often prohibitive cost of Western-type treatment?

It was decided to begin work in four areas, winning the confidence of the people and convincing them that they could achieve health cheaply. The scheme co-operated with Government, attempted a "family-doctor" system, providing modern treatment for each family while maintaining a link with the herbal practitioner, and trained interns and nurses in concepts of comprehensive care.

"Family folders" were constructed, giving a full health picture for each member of every family. Then a varied programme of service was given along the usual lines: curative medicine, maternal and child health care, nutrition advice, environmental sanitation and immunization schedules.

The programme was to be evaluated after 1, 2½ and 5 years, by a study of the folders to see if infant and maternal mortality rates were falling, and children's weights were rising, and by recording whether doctors and nurses became more enthusiastic over the survey.

The communities cared for were at Field Ganj in a high-population-density area of the city, and Jamalpur, Lalton Kalan and Narangwal in the surrounding countryside. The latter two centres had numerous branch clinics.

Dr. Dillon headed the scheme, and inspired a team of doctors and health visitors.

The interns—students who had passed their final examinations but had not yet taken their degrees—learnt to treat patients using simple equipment and doing their own laboratory tests. They carried out village surveys, filling up the folders with details of each family, and making sketch maps of the area.

Student nurses learnt how to teach the essentials of health effectively, and gained experience in giving immunizations. And the village dais (traditional midwives) listened to lectures and worked for State examinations.

By 1973 38,000 people were being fully cared for at simple level, and health teams had visited every family at least quarterly. But in some directions progress was very slow. Open tuberculosis was not regarded seriously by ordinary people, and family planning advice was often ignored.

Such schemes as the one at Ludhiana are of great value in training medical and nursing students and graduates, but because it is a training programme for a medical and nursing school, the level of staffing and the cost of the scheme are far greater than could be afforded for the country as a whole.

But other mission hospitals, impressed by the experience which Ludhiana has gained, are asking for help in starting their own schemes. In response, the Medical College sends trained staff to give advice.

The Aroles

Drs. Raj and Mabelle Arole, by contrast, set out to establish a community health service that was self-supporting.[5] This was, however, only one of their aims.

They had qualified together from the Christian Medical College at Vellore, South India in 1959, and worked in the village of Vadala for 5 years. But then they said "We're treating only the patients who come to our doorstep. What about the thousands of others?" They wanted to find another way to meet rural India's health needs.

After study in North America they returned with clear aims in their minds. They were going to find a place which was really poor—as poor as anywhere in India. It must be a place where there were no Christians and no Christian work. And the people there must be desperately anxious for medical care.

They settled on Jamkhed, a village of 6–7,000 people in Maharastra state in Western India, 300 miles from Bombay. Jamkhed lies in a district where in recent years the rains have been very scarce and famine has been severe. There were no Christians there, and the people wanted help.

Drs. Raj and Mabelle laid down strict conditions. The villagers would have to take over financial responsibility for the scheme within five years. The only money available, given by American churches, was going to be used to begin the work, but they and the Government would have to carry it on.

Land was quickly given for their use, and also a bare building with no facilities, for the health team to live in. Work began in January 1971 and for three months the doctors were busy indeed with curative care.

When those from other villages asked for help too, Dr. Raj and his wife said "We can't visit you if you haven't got a proper road." So the people worked hard to clear a way. In the same way the doctors insisted—"If you want your children immunized, you must collect 90% of all the little children in the village." 95% came.

So it was also with the feeding campaigns for toddlers: the people themselves must provide fuel for the kitchens and cook the food.

The Aroles have other clear lines of strategy. First each skilled person must delegate as much of his work as he possibly can. The doctors hand over much of the diagnosis and treatment—including suturing wounds and extracting teeth—to the nurses. The nurses delegate to more simply-trained nurse-midwives. These again give as much responsibility as possible to village health workers who are illiterate but nevertheless most effective in persuading neighbouring women to accept family-planning advice.

The doctors stress prevention, and are determined that 70% of their time must be spent in preventive work, and only 30% in curative care.

As in other community health schemes, care of children under five years old is a major concern. In 30 villages the mortality in this age group has been cut by 50%, and every village sets aside two acres of land to grow high protein food for toddlers.

Family-planning is likewise greatly emphasized. The aim is to reduce the birth-rate from 40 per thousand to 30 per thousand. Excellent puppet shows drive home the need for smaller families.

Tuberculosis, with 15 people infected out of every 1,000, and leprosy with 12 sufferers among every 1,000, are tackled energetically. Careful surveys are done to find all who need treatment. Leprosy patients are treated in ordinary clinics along with everyone else, and the Aroles make a point of putting their hands on each of them to dispel the exaggerated fears of contagion which other people have.

Each of the leprosy patients is given six fast-breeding goats. He drinks the milk and returns some of the kids to help others.

The doctors have wide interests; wells are dug, using a well-boring scheme, on the understanding that a farmer who gains a well will be generous in return. Pumps are given to villages, and tractors are rented.

The Aroles have a hospital but they keep it small, just 24 beds, sufficient to deal with emergencies. Much of the non-urgent surgical work is sent on to the Salvation Army hospital, 50 miles away.

Pat Nickson, a visiting missionary nurse, spoke of the Christian witness of the whole project. "Each person on the team," she wrote, "shewed the love of Christ." The lighted cross on the hospital, which can be seen 15 miles away, is a reminder, says Dr. Mabelle, "of the power of God in Christ."

An experiment in Bangladesh

Bangladesh is one of the neediest countries in the world—the most crowded of all (if one excepts very small places like Hong Kong), with 1,350 people to the square mile compared with 600 to the square mile in Britain. And this population is likely to double itself in the next 20 years.

The Bangladeshi suffered severely from civil war at the time of the partition of Pakistan in December 1971. Disastrous cyclones make hundreds of thousands homeless. The many rivers overflow their banks with widespread flooding. And the country's jute industry is cut off from its long established factories, which are now in India on the other side of the border.

To try and meet Bangladesh's most urgent health needs over a small area, a little group of doctors started work at Savar, about ten miles from the capital, Dacca. This was not a Christian venture, but indeed undertaken in a sacrificial, caring way.[6]

The doctors were determined not to be involved in hospital care, but to keep the project at health centre level. While a permanent building was going up, they started work in corrugated iron huts on the muddy building site.

They aimed to show that comprehensive care could be given to a whole unit of population with nobody neglected or overlooked. They began by collecting statistics, village by village, using high school students who worked as volunteers in the evenings and at week-ends.

A central clinic was started with small branch clinics in six villages; these are the forerunners of 13 village sub-centres, each of which will have its full-time staff of para-medics (medical auxiliaries), helped by local volunteers.

A determined attempt has been made to make the scheme largely self-supporting through health insurance. Each family pays 2 taka (10p, $0.20) a month, which does not cover the cost, but helps greatly. Most families can afford this. The family is then entitled to out-patient treatment, emergency care, drugs and immunizations.

Much house-to-house visiting was needed to win support for the scheme, but by 1974 over 2,000 families were contributing regularly.

Family-planning is an urgent need. In some villages volunteer family-planning counsellors deliver pills to the homes themselves, thus reducing the number of women who drop out of the scheme. A small charge of TK 0.25 a month (1½p, $0.03) is made for the pills, so that mothers can choose to use the service rather than having it pressed upon them.

The Savar staff have plenty of good ideas. They want to mobilize the women of the country as a huge force for rural development. As a small first step, 35% of their staff are women, a very unusual proportion in that country, and the girl paramedicals are given bicycles to ride.

After a year's work the doctors were convinced that the biggest health need in Bangladesh was more and better food. So they decided that all the staff, doctors included, would spend an hour each morning cultivating in the fields, to prove that they did not merely talk about better crops, but were helping to grow them too.

They want to see "para-agros", as well as paramedicals; that is, experts on farming who work at simple level, having received practical training locally.

Like the Chinese, they know the value of human night-soil (which produces combustible gas too), and hen manure, as fertilizers. They also encourage the full use of fish ponds.

And then what to do about the poverty which cripples the health of so many people? More chances for employment are essential. So Savar started to train girls to use sewing machines in order to make children's clothes. But material is expensive and jute handicrafts are being tried instead. Pottery made at a local co-operative is marketed in the main clinic.

Plenty of difficulties

Encouraging as accounts of such projects are, much trial and error, failure and heartache go into the establishment of them. John Sibley, surgeon transformed into medical project director of a community health scheme on the island of Kojedo, Korea, writes honestly and movingly about his difficulties.[7]

Traditionally trained missionary doctors in overseas countries should be made aware, says Sibley, that there is a better way of providing health care than through institutions alone, but "this is extremely hard to do."

It took him six years of exposure to the problem before he would even consider the thought that there might be a better way than through the hospital.

When he finally agreed that a different kind of medical care was needed, he spent six months studying community medicine in different countries—a short enough time, as he says, for a plastic surgeon to train himself in public health, paediatrics, administration and personnel management.

He was pointed in the right direction then, as he admits, but many troubles lay ahead. One of the greatest was the change from being an acknowledged expert in his field to being an authority on virtually nothing. And there were so many problems to solve.

What, he asked himself, is the minimum needed to set up a competent accounting system—answer; an American high-school graduate on the island, and a certified accountant 300 miles (480 km) away. What does one do when the only good refrigerator breaks down when full of vaccine—"our somewhat inadequate answer; shake it hard and pray." Where can one buy a cheap portable X-ray? How do you set up a system of self-support? Questions and posers swamp the doctor in charge.

And so John Sibley urges—keep the project as small as possible. This is vital for an additional reason. It is easy to talk of "community involvement," "improved health", and "health education"; and these terms are simple to understand: but they are fantastically difficult to put into practice. Each phrase is a major project in itself, and so the scope of the enterprise must be limited if the doctor is to cope at all.

Sibley goes on to emphasize that what has succeeded in one country may not work in another. Doctors may delegate certain forms of treatment to nurses in India, but this is forbidden by law in Korea. He thought that simple health care would be popular in a somewhat remote village in Kojedo island, but a granny there was disappointed that its scope was so limited.

He had hoped for full government co-operation in his health programme, already endorsed by the Ministry of Health, all the more as the local government health clinic stressed the importance of immunization programmes such as the one that he was promoting; but the development of such co-operation met with many initial difficulties and misunderstandings.

And most of all the project leaders had underestimated the difficulty of asking a Korean doctor to work in such an isolated spot, with consequent loss of chances of promotion, and the impossibility of educating his children locally. There was only one applicant in two years.

He realized slowly that Korea was not yet ripe for a "broad community-centred health programme". "Community self-help projects" needed much education on the importance of co-operation and mutual trust outside family circles. "Co-operation with Government" could only be built up slowly, by much patience and steady mutual understanding. "Self-support" would only come when progress had been made in the above directions. And so they settled down to steady education of the people on what the health needs were and how they should be met, while still keeping all their other goals in view.

Bit by bit "the wheels began to grip, rather than to spin," as Sibley says, and after three years of work he could write of a typical spring day at Kojedo:

". . . the waiting room already has a small gathering of men, women and children waiting for the clinic to open, and they join us there at morning worship, led by Mr. Lee, the business manager. By 9 o'clock the morning clinic begins, run by Dr. Kim with the OPD nurse, the lab and X-ray technician and six aides, including a clerk, pharmacist and laboratory assistant. As the car is being loaded for the outreach and home-visiting trip to a cluster of villages 10 kilometres to the north, Dr. Adams and an aide walk past on their way to the pier, for the ride across the strait to Chil Chun Island and a well-baby clinic in the village of Mulan.

"More patients arrive on the bus from the township to the north, and the generator is started for the first of a series of X-rays, its muffled clamour soon joined by that of the tiller at work in the field by the well. In the waiting room an aide is giving an enthusiastic lecture on the importance of family-planning, while in the office the Peace Corps volunteer is reviewing TB patient cards with an aide, in preparation for home-visiting that afternoon.

"While I am checking the four patients admitted to the in-patient building, an aide informs me that Dr. Kim has a patient he wants me to see. A student has a laceration of her lower lip and needs suturing . . .

"Large gaps still remain—but the project is taking shape."

References   Chapter 6

1. Stanfield, J. Paget ed. "Recent Approaches to Malnutrition in Uganda," section VIII. Reprinted from the *Journal of Tropical Pediatrics and Environmental Child Health,* **17**, 1971, p. 67.
2. Proposal for the Community Health Programme of Christian Medical College, Punjab. (mimeo) *circa* 1972, and annual reports of the Programme for 1972 and 1973.
3. Bryant, John, *Health and the Developing World,* Cornell, Ithaca N.Y., 1969, p. 91.
4. Morley, David. *Pediatric Priorities in the Developing World,* Butterworths, London, 1973, p. 4.
5. Mook, Jane Day. AD Magazine of United Church in USA: reprinted in *Vellore Newsletter*, No. 58, March 1974 (36 St. George's Street, Winchester).
6. Report of Gonshasthya Kendra, P.O. Nayahat, District Dacca, No. 4, July 1973–April 1974.
7. Sibley, John R. *Community Health—Progress and Problems.* Kojedo Project. Christian Medical Commission Annual Meeting, Nemi (Rome) 1971, Pub. CMC Geneva.

Chapter 7

LESSONS FROM CHINA

"Solve the problems facing the masses—food, shelter and clothing —sickness and hygiene . . . ; in short, all the practical problems of the masses' everyday life should claim our attention. If we attend to the problems . . . they will rally round us and give us their warm support." So wrote Mao Tse-tung in 1934.[1]

It is impossible to study health care in developing countries adequately without trying to understand the remarkable achievements that China has made in this field in the last 25 years.

It is itself a developing country, with four-fifths of its population of 800 million people living in rural areas and supporting themselves by farming.[2]

In similar countries in Asia there are relatively few highly qualified doctors and these mainly concentrated in the towns, very scanty rural health services, and widely prevalent infectious diseases. China now has about 1 million barefoot doctors and the like who are evenly distributed throughout the country, has succeeded in eradicating smallpox, leprosy, plague and cholera, and has brought tuberculosis and bilharzia under control.

Up to 1949 China had the same health imbalances and defects as are seen in neighbouring countries today. But in 1950 four principles were laid down:

Health care must serve the common people
Priority must be given to preventing disease
Western and traditional medicine must be combined
Health campaigns must be combined with other mass campaigns[3]

During the next 15 years there were periods when emphasis was laid on the development of urban areas, and on excellence in medical research and training.

But in the Cultural Revolution of 1966, it was determined that rural areas must be especially cared for; "in health, place stress on the countryside," said Mao.[4]

City workers were sent to join rural mobile medical teams: barefoot doctors were trained in large numbers, and co-operative medical care was established, based on the commune.

Using traditional doctors

Records of traditional Chinese medicine go back to 1700 BC. Its philosophy rests on the need for balance and harmony between man and nature. When a man falls ill, his body's balance is disturbed.

By detailed questioning and feeling the pulse, the traditional doctor can tell which part of the body is at fault. He may treat the patient by herbal remedies such as herbal teas, or by moxibustion, acupuncture and exercises.

Moxibustion consists in burning the moxa herb close to the skin: the local heat benefits rheumatic pain.[5] By acupuncture, at present a subject of great interest, is meant the introduction of long fine needles into certain definite parts of the body for the treatment of pain, or in recent years, to produce anaesthesia before surgical operations.

Hundreds of herbs are used medicinally by the half-million traditional practitioners who are now incorporated into the country's health service, to serve in outpatient clinics and rural health centres.[6]

They provide emotional support to patients by being generous in the time they give for treatment:[7] they can relieve chronic rheumatic troubles in particular: and their remedies give symptomatic relief in common complaints such as virus infections, which run their course without needing powerful drugs to control them.

Herbal treatment is popular because familiar, and is both simple and cheap. Western-trained and traditional doctors work side by side in clinics, the old methods acting as a bridge to introduce the peasant to modern ways of preventing and treating disease.

The barefoot doctor

"Soon after lunch people began coming to the health station in Sun village. A woman production leader came in holding one hand over her ear. A young barefoot doctor examined her and said it was infection of the outer ear. He weighed out some dried dandelions and honeysuckles, wrapped them in a piece of paper, and handed them to her with instructions to make a broth from them. She had just gone when an elderly woman who suffers from chronic high blood pressure came in for her regular injection. A mischievous-looking boy dashed in and stood very still in front of the medicine chest. The barefoot doctor changed the dressing for a boil on his head. 'All right, scoot!' he said, giving him a pat on the behind as he finished. The boy ran off.

"It all seemed to be happening in one big family . . . it wasn't just that the patients did not have to register or pay any fee. What is more impressive is their complete trust in the doctors and the doctors' warm informality with them."[8]

The title "barefoot doctor" is a misnomer. They often—perhaps usually—wear shoes,[9] and are not doctors in the Western sense. As David Bonavia says,[10] they are something of a cross between public health inspector and district nurse. Many of them are women.

They are usually young peasants who spend part of their time in farm work, and part in giving health care. They are intelligent and educated to junior middle school level.

Barefoot doctors spend four months receiving basic training, learning how to recognize the symptoms of common diseases, and how to treat them by both traditional and western methods.

Then they go home with a box of simple medical supplies. When there is not so much to do on the farm they come back for a second four-month course, and so on for three years, by which time they can recognize seventy-five common diseases. They do not receive any certificate at the end of this time, as their education is considered to be life-long.

Much time is given to preventive work, such as immunization campaigns, promotion of family-planning, eradication of flies and mosquitoes, and ensuring a clean water supply.

They do not get paid specially for their health work; this[11] counts for points in their wages, in the same way as their farming work.

Their opposite numbers in industry are the "worker doctors", employed in factory jobs with a special concern for industrial health.

Barefoot doctors are part of a pyramid of health staff. Below them are family health workers and "Red Guard doctors", who give first-aid and help with public health campaigns. Above them are doctors of western medicine and fully-trained nurses.[12]

Health care at barefoot doctor level is financed by small insurance contributions. Each person in a production brigade, which is the local community of about 700 people, pays 20p ($0.40) a year to the co-operative medical scheme, and brigade funds add an equal amount.[2]

The conquest of epidemic disease

In 1950 smallpox, tuberculosis and cholera were widespread.The eradication in whole or in part of these and other infectious and parasitic diseases is a triumph of planning and co-ordinated effort.

The secrets of success have been, first, that prevention was given priority over cure, not merely on paper but in practice. Then, as already stated, health campaigns were co-ordinated with other mass efforts, such as improvement of farming methods, or provision of better irrigation. Full use was made of the abundant labour available. And lastly, nothing was done without the full agreement of the people at every level, the so-called "mass-line".

The phrase "mass-line" describes a new line of policy which has been fully accepted and adopted by the masses of the people. China's planning rests on the belief that ordinary people can understand and solve complicated problems if these are fully explained and the right encouragement is given.

So a new plan brought out by the leaders is discussed at every level of the community, and modified as necessary in response to objections. Only after long study periods have produced general agreement can the new proposals be carried out.

In health matters, naturally all this study and discussion is a very effective means of health education. The usual films, posters and lectures are used, and then there are group discussions, first for understanding and then for action.

The fight against schistosomiasis (bilharzia infection) gives an example of the results that are achieved, once the mass-line is accepted.

The disease is caused in China by the worm schistosoma japonicum. This develops in a freshwater snail, and then invades humans wading in water, causing painful inflammation in the bladder and rectum, which may result in serious ill-health and premature death.

The problem which has defeated many other countries is how to with kill all the snails and cure everyone who has been infected.

China has one advantage in that these particular snails only live at the water's edge, instead of being under-water snails as in other countries. If they are buried beneath the surface of the water, they die.

So thousands of peasants diverted water from irrigation ditches, sliced off the earth at the sides of the ditches, as it was here that the snails were found, and dumped this earth at the bottom of the ditch, covering it with fresh soil. Then the ditch could be filled again with water, or even levelled up with earth and a new ditch dug.

All this was an opportunity to improve irrigation and at the same time to apply lime and fertilizer to the fields.

The community was now checked by barefoot doctors to find all those infected, so that they might have a course of intravenous injections.

And, most important, careful supervision was continued afterwards. Peasants are examined yearly for schistosomes, and recurring cases are treated[13]

Such a campaign is not an isolated drive against one disease, as say leprosy control may sometimes appear. It is part of a broad based struggle for better health, which began with an attack on the "four pests", originally rats, flies, mosquitoes, and sparrows. Sparrows were found to keep down insect-pests in the fields and so bed-bugs were substituted as a target. Now it is said to be rare to find flies or mosquitoes in any village.

In the early days everyone had a quota of pests to be killed, and I feel much sympathy for the university professor who came in tears to his colleagues to buy a few rats to make up his allotted quota!

Each week there is a day for cleaning the streets and disposing of rubbish. Office workers turn out with the rest and do their share of sweeping.

Changing the elitist image

One of the attractive features of recent Chinese medical history is the new attitude of fully-trained doctors. In earlier days they were mainly found in the cities, being orientated to hospital medicine, private practice and prestige.

Now, not without a big struggle and perhaps only with partial success, they are spending time in rural areas, becoming interested in simple preventive measures, and working side by side with auxiliaries.

This has been achieved largely through mobile medical teams. Urban doctors go to the countryside to treat patients and up-grade the health services. The President of the Chinese Academy of Medicine, Dr. Huang Chia-ssu, describes[14] how he operated in a rural clinic, when "one patient with acute intestinal obstruction had to have a section of his intestine removed. Ordinarily this would only be done in a regular hospital, but there was no time to lose. Dr. Tseng Hsien-Chiu, head of the surgical department of Peking Union Hospital, and I worked together on the surgery, which took 4 hours. With good post-operative care, the patient soon recovered." Dr. Huang Chia-ssu, who is a well-known thoracic surgeon, also gave mass treatment for trachoma, experimented on the best ways to stop flies breeding in latrines, and established a health workers training course in a farm-school.

The city doctors lived with the peasants and there is a pleasant picture of Dr. Hsu Chia-yu, medical specialist in Shanghai, living in the home of a barefoot doctor and adapting to the rough surroundings and simple food. The two men have to share one bed at night with the same pillow, and they lie awake for a time, discussing the patients they have seen during the day and talking about their hopes for society.[15]

Medical graduates of the future will make these adjustments much more easily. They will start their course having been recommended as suitable students by their communes, and after having spent an adequate time in productive work, like everyone else. Their course has been shortened so that more can be trained.

They have to devote nine months of the three years' curriculum to practical medical work in the countryside with their teachers, as members of mobile medical teams. By day the students see a wide range of clinical conditions, and in the evening they have lectures in the local primary school. They are trained on the spot in preventive medicine, and both students and lecturers do regular manual work in the fields or on the roads.

Maybe later on the three year course will be lengthened, and post-graduate training given, but for the present the need is for plenty of graduates with practical experience.

Doctors in mental hospitals are equally free from professional aloofness. They share in the patients' work and recreation, act in plays with them, and make the running of the hospital a joint patient/staff affair. By visits to each patient's home and place of work before he is discharged, they make sure that he is given every chance, by support and encouragement, to keep well after he leaves hospital.

Would the methods of China work elsewhere?

It is hard to know how far China's achievements could be copied in other developing countries, and especially in small church-related health projects.

It is tempting to wish that in all Third World countries we could see qualified doctors who were willing to work in rural areas on the prevention of disease, and auxiliaries like the barefoot doctors who would give a neighbourhood service for every fifty families in remote areas, as well as communities which would fight epidemic disease and at the same time improve food production. But the difficulties of reproducing such successes are indeed very great. Nevertheless China has important lessons to teach us about future patterns of Christian health care elsewhere.

Missionary doctors and nurses in China left a great record of devotion and self-sacrifice. Yet we can now see weaknesses in their approach which should be avoided in future.

Victor Hayward has pointed out that, much as such work was appreciated, it was carried out wholly on Western lines without any appreciation of what was valuable in traditional medicine. Medical graduates became a Westernized élite, hospital treatment was made available for the few instead of disease prevention for the many, and the Church as a whole was not encouraged to think seriously about political issues and social responsibility.[16]

These mistakes must not be repeated. Yet as Hayward says, the changes in China only occurred after a revolution in which some two million lives were lost—with the further and graver Cultural Revolution to follow in 1966 to 1969. (Hayward warns that this loss of life must be seen in proportion. Two million is 0·3% of the population. And the severity of these terrible upheavals must in fairness be compared in numerical proportion with the religious wars of Europe in past centuries, and the results compared also.)[17]

Further, and more important still, perhaps, Chinese society is now wholly "directed".[18] Everyone has to believe the same teachings, no one must step out of the "correct line", no one can choose where he will live or work.

But the Christian cannot in any way surrender the privilege of loving and obeying God with all his heart, and then living a life of spiritual freedom, growing in personal responsibility, and looking to the day when he will see God face to face.

Not only is there this insuperable barrier to a full adoption of the Chinese health care system, but China has assets which perhaps no other country possesses: an immense reserve of ample manpower for labour, a closed economy which is effective because of the country's size, and a scheme of traditional medicine older and more developed than probably anywhere in the world.

Yet if these achievements cannot be fully copied,[19] the precepts that China laid down in 1950—be concerned for the common people, put prevention before cure, find a place for traditional medicine, and combine health care with development in other directions—all these deserve to be underlined and fully adopted in Christian medical work today.

And equally the Chinese concept of a Western-trained doctor as humble, accustomed to working in a health team, ready to share in practical community work, and full of a love for country life and country people—how attractive and desirable this seems.

So when we study the barefoot doctor again, the medical auxiliary whom in one form or another all countries need, and mark his (or her) assured place in the "flattened pyramid" of health workers, bringing preventive and curative medicine and health education to a small community where he is known and trusted, we must wish to see his counterpart given an honoured place in all Christian health endeavour, not to say in health care everywhere.

References **Chapter 7**

1. *Health care in China: an introduction*, Christian Medical Commission, Geneva 1974, p. 17.
2. Smith, Tony. *The Times*, June 29 1974.
3. *Health Care in China*, p. 18.
4. ibid, p. 26.
5. Smith, A. J. *British Medical Journal*, 1974, **2,** pp. 367–370.
6. *Health Care in China*, pp. 88–91.
7. Rifkin, Susan and Kaplinsky, Raphael. *Health Strategy and Development Planning—China*, Tropical Child Health Unit, Institute of Child Health, London.
8. *Health Care in China*, p. 48.
9. Sidel, V. *Update*, October 1974, p. 833.
10. *The Times*, July 17 1975.
11. Li, Victor H. *China Quarterly*, 1974, **59,** p. 566.
12. *Health Care in China*, p. 107.
13. ibid, pp. 67–71.
14. ibid, p. 115.
15. Sidel, V. op cit.
16. Hayward, Victor. *Christians and China*, Christian Journals Ltd, Belfast, 1974, p. 33.
17. ibid, pp. 111–113.
18. ibid, p. 115.
19. Smith, A. J. and Adey, Evelyn M., *British Medical Journal*, 1974, **2,** pp. 603–605.

Chapter 8

THE PLACE OF THE HOSPITAL

"This afternoon I went to see a patient at the hospital.
From ward to ward I walked, through that city of suffering, sensing the tragedies hardly concealed by the brightly painted walls and the flower bordered lawns.
I had to go through a ward: I walked on tiptoe, hunting for my patient.
My eyes passed quickly and discreetly over the sick, as one touches a wound delicately to avoid hurting.
I felt uncomfortable,
Like the uninitiated traveller lost in a mysterious temple . . ."

Michel Quoist.
Prayers of Life, Gill & Son, Dublin, 1963.

Hospitals impress the visitor deeply with a sense of the suffering which is borne there, the crises of birth and death which occur in them, the contrast between the tension of acute illness and the relaxed look of the patient well on the way to recovery, the youth and freshness of the nurses and the lined faces of those who will never recover.

No wonder they are places which have very special importance in the life of any community. And mission hospitals, each founded by a doctor with unusual gifts of skill and energy, stamped with his personality, and remembered by church leaders as the places where their parents were nursed and their children born, are looked up to as an integral part of the life of the church and a cause of pride and thankfulness.

Indeed, in cases of serious illness, the hospital reigns supreme. If the patient has a strangulated hernia, if a woman is admitted in obstructed labour and needs a Caesarean section, if a boy is brought after several days of unexplained fever, or a baby with meningitis needs skilled treatment, there is only one place for them, and that is a hospital.

But today the church hospital faces big problems. Perhaps when it was founded, it was the only hospital in the town or district. Now there is a Government hospital, maybe even a medical school, only a few miles away. And whereas the founder was the one western-trained doctor for a hundred miles around, now there are many doctors within a short distance. No wonder the staff ask themselves what is their special contribution today.

The question of expense

And the cost of maintaining the hospital is a constant anxiety. In Britain in mid-1975 treatment in a National Health Service hospital bed cost over £30 ($60) a day—say over £10,000 ($20,000) a year.[1] In India or Africa the daily figure is smaller, but still beyond the ability of the poorest part of the population to pay. The tension between having to treat the better-off, so as to balance the budget, and finding ways of caring for those who need help but cannot afford it, is a constant source of pain for the medical missionary, most of all in his early years.

Treating those who are nearest

Again, the hospital tends to treat mainly those who live near to it. Mulago Hospital in Kampala is the specialized reference hospital for the whole of Uganda. But in 1964 90% of all the sick children treated there, and 98% of all mothers who had babies there, came from Mengo district, the administrative area immediately around the hospital.[2]

Maurice King has pointed out that if we plot on a map the distance that patients live from the hospital, we find that those who are 2 km (1 mile) away attend on average five times a year, while from homes 8 km (5 miles) distant, there is only one attendance a year.[3] This is understandable where transport is difficult and many patients come on foot, but it underlines the limited influence of the hospital on the community.

Do all hospital patients need that standard of care?

In a developing country at least, many of the conditions treated in hospital ought never to have arrived there: they are illnesses that should have been treated elsewhere.

Helen Gideon studied the pattern of disease in 1,032 out-patients and 681 in-patients in 8 mission hospitals in India.[4] She concluded that 48% of the out-patients and 44% of the in-patients would never have had to come to hospital if they had been treated or protected at an earlier stage by a medical auxiliary.

Those with the highest incidence of preventable disease were the children under 5. 80% of the out-patients and 67% of the in-patients in this age group had illnesses which could easily have been avoided.

Sister O'Keeffe did a similar study at Mtendere Hospital in Zambia, a hospital of 70 beds with one doctor and three nursing sisters.[5] 40% of the patients were children under 5.

She discovered that 54% of hospital attenders had mild conditions which did not need hospital care at all. The majority of patients coming for help lived within 10 miles. And on the whole the hospital was used for the need of the moment by those who lived near it.

At the same time, 65% of children in a primary school in the same area were suffering from bilharzial infection, and 77% of a group of toddlers over the age of 1 year had not been immunized against any infectious disease.

She concluded, in short, that the bulk of disease seen both in hospital and in the population around was *community* disease. But the hospital met the needs of individuals only. What was the use, she asked, of giving expensive treatment to cure a patient's bilharzia, when 50% of the population depend on a bilharzia-infected source for their water supply?

Treat the community

She urged that better health must start in the community, with medical workers joining with agriculturists, community development officers, water affairs experts and school teachers in order to attack the main problems.

In addition, the people in each village must themselves shoulder responsibility for achieving a much higher standard of health. Then the hospital will have its right but limited place in the community.

David Morley, writing in a similar style, stresses that the hospital should actively improve the health of the community around it.[6] It could do this by setting up health centres, and then by training the community to help itself—a recurring theme of many health planners. Using volunteer groups of all kinds and village medical aides, the hospital would have a broad base of human support.

The picture thus comes clearer. A church hospital in a developing country should ideally be the central point of a net-work of health centres or aid posts which are active in prevention and treatment. As far as possible only those patients would be referred to hospital who needed treatment for surgical emergencies, or special X-ray and laboratory investigations, or skilled nursing for serious illness.

If there were a Government hospital within fairly easy reach by bus, to which non-urgent surgical problems could be referred, then the church hospital might remain quite small. There are about 770 hospitals in the United Kingdom each with less than 50 beds.[7] Admittedly major surgery is not done in them, because surgical facilities are so quickly available elsewhere. But if a church hospital were dealing mainly with patients referred from village clinics it could do a great deal with relatively few beds, under 50 perhaps, provided that it had the essential facilities of operating theatre, laboratory, X-ray unit, and pharmacy. And provided too that there was access to a not-too-distant Government hospital with a wider range of services.

The second function of a church hospital should be to teach—to train as many people as possible at different levels. It could train nurses or medical aides at whatever simple level the Government would authorize, perhaps affiliating to another hospital to make sure that a sufficiently varied practical experience was gained.

Besides this formal training, the whole hospital staff should become community orientated by frank discussions and visits to other units, to quote David Morley again. And all members of staff, including cleaners and ward attendants, need training in simple health education, so that everyone to whom the patient turns for advice will give the same clear answer on a few leading health topics.

It does look indeed as if the special characteristic of the Christian hospital or church hospital should be that it is a community hospital, part of the life of the community in which it is placed. It would not compete with the bigger state or university institutions nearby, but it would have its own particular educative function that would be of the greatest value.

A school for society

Michael Wilson calls a hospital a living learning arena, a school for society, where attitudes to illness, health, ageing and death are taught. Patients, their families and all staff must learn and feed back into society what it means to be human, both in illness and during the time of growing older.[8]

In this "learning for life" experience which a hospital provides, the place of the family is important indeed. Mission hospitals in the past have often struggled to keep the family out. Relatives of patients were banished from the ward during the main working hours. But the rules began to be relaxed first of all in the children's ward, so that mothers might have plenty of time to feed their babies, and to "pot" them individually, cutting down the risk of cross-infection by diarrhoeal disease.

Doctors and nurses soon saw how much the mothers could gain during these days in hospital, just by watching, listening to advice, and learning new skills.

Now at the Mental Health Centre in Vellore, S. India, one or two members of the family stay with the patient throughout the treatment programme, without any restriction. They bring patients for electro-convulsive treatment and look after them during the recovery time. They have group meetings, supervised by staff, where they discuss mental illness and gain fresh attitudes to it.

The therapists talk to the relatives about the rest of the family at home, discovering where the tensions are and trying to restore a happy balance of relationships.

Patients feel happier when they have their relatives with them, and find that the hospital does not feel so strange. When the time comes for discharge, the relatives have the ongoing treatment explained to them, and they are asked to keep in touch with the staff and return for follow-up if possible.

The patient does not experience an abrupt change from hospital to home, as the same relatives are with him in both places, helping him to improve. And what the little group of two or three has learnt in the hospital soon becomes common knowledge throughout their community, changing attitudes to mental illness.[9]

If relatives can "learn for life" in the hospital, so can the patient. But first of all he must be treated as a real person, someone with human dignity, whose fears and problems call for respect and understanding.

Psychiatrists can teach us so much by their "whole-man" attitude to patients, and John Bavington, in another Mental Health Centre, this time in Peshawar in Pakistan, describes his approach.[10]

"It sometimes happens", he writes, "that a disturbed person is brought to our hospital bound or having to be held down by several strong people. I have often found that by taking the person alone into a quiet room, his violence and the need for physical restraint are removed. What has happened? Previously his disturbed behaviour, which may have been due to severe anxiety, was met with a hostility which created further anxiety, and hence more disturbance. In the different setting, we were seeking to communicate a sense of reassurance which would free him from having to behave like a frightened animal. This communication is a matter of attitude rather than words, and is an important part of a helpful therapeutic relationship."

"Recently I was asked", he continues, "to visit a man who for weeks had been shouting at night and abusing and disturbing the neighbours and making his relatives' lives impossible. They expected that we would come and give him some injection to quiet him and then take him to our hospital by force. He perhaps also expected this, and was obviously very anxious and resistant when we met him.

"We sat down and talked quietly with him, and left saying that we would call again the following day. We did call, but again he did not want to accompany us to hospital or take our medicines. However, on the third day his family thought it was quite miraculous when he quietly agreed to come to the hospital. Somehow we had got through to him and relieved his suspicion enough for him to be able to accept our help.

"I believe this principle is very much applicable to our missionary task," he goes on. "A community of Christians really incarnating the spirit of the Gospel would be a potent medium, since it is very difficult to resist such indirect approaches. They somehow by-pass conscious intellectual defences and do their quiet work at the level of the heart."

In an atmosphere of friendliness and acceptance patients may be able to bring out the fears and worries which weigh heavily upon them. In Mengo Hospital a patient was admitted after a fall from a horse. Fractured ribs had caused a haemothorax—bleeding outside the lung. This was dealt with but the patient remained anxious and depressed. "You look very worried," said an African nurse gently, "I think you need my Jesus", and comforted her with Bible promises. It turned out that a friend of the patient had had a similar accident, dying on the third day, and so the patient was dreading the same outcome. She was reassured and made a complete recovery.

Again the patient can be encouraged, by the renewed confidence which he feels, to take as much responsibility as possible for the management of his own illness—the goal which Ivan Illich rightly considers as so important. Sedatives and drugs for relieving minor pains will then be used only for an acute episode which is soon over.

In some psychiatric hospitals it has been realized that the total atmosphere of the hospital has a powerful influence on the patient for good or ill, and the "therapeutic community" has been introduced to use the institutional setting to the best advantage.

Caroline Currer at the Mental Health Centre in Peshawar describes how such a community works.[11] Communication between members of staff and between staff and patients, she explains, is encouraged as fully as possible, and daily meetings are held for this purpose. All problems of daily work, treatment and relationships are discussed at these times.

The "authority pyramid is flattened", that is to say, such free communication produces new relationships in which every member of the staff, however junior, and every patient is considered as having an important contribution to make, and so positions of authority are much modified.

Again throughout the day every opportunity is taken to encourage a patient to take part in the life of the unit, and be self-reliant.

Of course the problems faced, the pressure of work, and the demands on the staff will differ greatly in a general hospital from those of a mental health unit, and frequent long meetings with all patients joining in would just not be possible in busy general wards. And in any case the therapeutic community is designed to meet disorders which are chiefly emotional.

But certain lessons from this approach can surely be widely applied. It is commonly said that "they never explained anything to me—the doctors always seemed too busy—when I asked the doctor why I was having this treatment, he seemed very annoyed." An authoritarian attitude in hospital deprives the patient of responsibility and reduces his dignity, creating something of a parent/child relationship.

Therefore much is gained by free exchanges of ideas and knowledge between staff and patients, by stimulating patients to understand and cope with their own illnesses and by encouraging junior members of staff, such as cleaners or wardmaids, to contribute their ideas and insights.

Would it seem a very unusual hospital if it were a place where the staff were constantly going outside to visit the community around, and the community was constantly coming inside in the form of relatives who would learn about their patients' illnesses? Where the doctors and nurses were very approachable and ready to listen and explain, the nurses always seeming to find a minute or two to sit by the bed and talk about anxieties or something not well understood? And where a junior wardmaid was listened to with respect, and decisions affecting the daily work of the staff were only undertaken after full discussion?

In fact these very characteristics are seen in many hospitals today—but maybe they need to be seen all together more often, and in a more wholehearted way.

Within such a hospital, each patient would grow in dignity and self-reliance, each family would be strengthened by the experience of illness, and the life of the whole community would be enriched.

References **Chapter 8**

1. *British Medical Journal*, 1975, **2,** p. 651.
2. *Mulago Hospital Admissions,* 1963 *and* 1964, P. J. S. Hamilton and M. Anderson (stencilled report).
3. King, Maurice. *Medical Care in Developing Countries*, Oxford University Press, London, 1966.
4. Gideon, Helen. *Contact* 17, October 1973, Christian Medical Commission, Geneva.
5. O'Keeffe, ibid.
6. Morley, David. *Contact* 20, April 1974, Christian Medical Commission, Geneva.
7. *The Times*, March 5 1973.
8. Wilson, Michael. *The Hospital a Place of Truth*, University of Birmingham, Institute for the Study of Worship, 1971.
9. Verghese, Abraham. *Journal of Christian Medical Association of India*, 1971, **46,** pp. 247–251.
10. Bavington, John. "Communication through Community", reprinted from *The Counsellor,* Journal of the Christian Study Centre, Rawalpindi, Pakistan, July–September 1972.
11. Currer, Caroline. "An attempt to Apply the 'Therapeutic Community' Approach to Treatment in Pakistan", Mission Hospital, Peshawar (mimeo 1975).

Chapter 9

WHAT KIND OF TRAINING?

Edward de Bono, in his book *The Use of Lateral Thinking*, tells the story of a merchant who was deeply in debt to an old and ugly money-lender. The money-lender wanted to marry the merchant's beautiful daughter, and proposed a plan.

A black and white pebble would be put in a bag and the girl would pick one out. If it were black she would become the wife and the debt would be cancelled. If white she would stay with her father, and the debt would still be cancelled. If she refused to pick out a pebble her father would be thrown into prison.

As the money-lender bent to pick the pebbles from the path, the girl saw that they were both black. What was she to do—refuse to take a pebble, sacrifice herself by taking a black one, or expose the trick? All would lead to disaster.

She was, as de Bono says, a "lateral thinker". Her mind swiftly produced an unusual solution to the problem. She put her hand in the bag, took out a pebble without looking at it, and fumblingly let it drop on the path, where it could not be distinguished from the others. "How silly of me", she said, "but still, we can tell which colour it was by looking at the one that is left." Of course this was black; the one taken was thought to be white (because the money-lender could not explain his trick) and she and her father were safe.[1]

Is West best?

Perhaps it is just this willingness to approach a problem in a novel way that we need in reviewing medical and nursing training in developing countries.

The principle in the past has been that what is best for Western countries is best everywhere. So medical students in Africa and Asia have been trained in the best models of European or North American medical schools, and where possible nursing training has been raised to the registered or graduate level achieved in the West.

The results have been firstly, great expense; the cost of training a doctor in Ethiopia (one of the poorest countries in the world) in 1972 was £14,000 ($28,000)[2] and in Nigeria in 1975 £30,000 ($60,000).[3] Furthermore, a doctor trained in a well-equipped modern hospital in a city understandably wishes to have access to similar facilities after graduation, and so he stays in city surroundings. Only 20% of the population of a developing country are in the cities, but this is where 80% of the doctors live, as David Morley has said. Or else the young doctor emigrates to an industrialized country, there to practise the kind of medicine to which he is used. In either case the 80% of his fellow countrymen who live in rural areas stand to lose heavily. Perhaps there will be one doctor for 50,000 of them, or maybe one to 100,000.

Again, the cost of employing registered nurses may be so great that church hospitals cannot afford to pay their salaries and have to consider closing their work, as has happened in Nigeria and Rwanda recently.

E. C. Long has urged "abandon any attempts to bring health care to rural areas by the extensive use of doctors and registered nurses, once and for all."[4] The most that will be achieved by training more doctors is that one just keeps level with the growth in population but never improves the doctor/patient ratio. And anyway their training is not fully appropriate at the present time to meet the main health problems which exist.

Begin with the family

So why not approach the problem from a different angle? Stanley Lang heard an African speaker at a World Health conference say that his country wanted "the polyvalent, multi-talented, available dedicated health person." Stanley comments "is this not the mother of the family?"[5]

Michael Church argues that ordinary people have a great capacity to keep themselves healthy. Villagers are actually surviving. How do they do it? Because they have resources of wisdom and experience on which to draw. And they are interested in the whole quality of life—with health as only one aspect of this.[6]

So should we not begin with a great respect for the family, and an earnest wish to understand the concepts which have guided generations of parents in the bringing up of their children?

Maybe we shall have to suggest changes in the way things are done—better infant feeding or better hygiene perhaps. But if so, we must not criticize the mother, who always does her best out of love for her child.

And any health education must reach the father too, as he is the decision maker, and the one who must give his consent. And it must have the blessing of the elders of the community, whose approval is vital: so there must be much discussion, patient explanation, and careful listening before new ideas are put into practice.

So everything begins with the family, which has such great strengths and powers of survival.

Recruiting the lay leaders and volunteers

The next step is the training of lay leaders. In Segbwema hospital in Sierra Leone, women who are already church leaders or married to church leaders come for a four-day course. They each bring a small child, and learn about the chief "toddler-killing" diseases and how to prevent them. They study family-planning, nutrition and the work of "under-fives" clinics. When they go back, (and 66 of them had been trained by 1974), they are installed by their chiefs as "nutritional leaders" and share their new knowledge with neighbouring families, each one at the same time training a helper to share her work.[7]

Drs. Rex and Jeanne Blumhagen are strong advocates for the training of "volunteer village health advisers" of this type. They argue that in countries like Bangladesh and Nepal it will be impossible in the near future to train the thousands of assistant nurses and midwives that are needed. Village leaders can and must share responsibility for health care.[8]

Suitable candidates are older women who are looked up to in the village, are willing to work, and are interested in new ideas. Pat Nickson describes their selection and training.

"At the start of the village health programme we decided that time should be spent in the villages, teaching and getting to know the people," she writes. "We supposed that by doing this, natural leaders would be noticed among the women. But experience showed that qualities of leadership, sympathetic understanding of people and honesty did not always go together, and we had to be more selective."

She and Sue Fry looked to see if any village women were interested in the correct way to conduct a normal delivery, and made a note of those who wanted to learn new methods. The opinions of a group of village women on the best choice of a local health worker helped them greatly too. They chose their students by a combination of their own impressions and this collective advice.

There were many difficulties to be faced by the new recruits, after the final selection had been made. Family feuds stopped village workers from looking after women on the opposite side. The workers had to stay in their own villages. And even a convinced village health worker could not always get new ideas over to a neighbour.

But still 17 women completed a basic health course on home hygiene and baby care, and 9 of them finished a second course on midwifery.

They gained practical experience in their own villages, using household equipment wherever possible, and were regularly supervised as long as the scheme lasted, with every effort being made to build up their status in the life of the village.[9]

The young man with some education who works for his community also makes an excellent volunteer. In Nepal these were chosen by the village council from among school teachers or farmers. They worked hard to convince villagers of the value of latrines and a clean water supply, though it took two years to win assent.

At Savar health centre near Dacca in Bangladesh young students attend weekly classes in health for three months, and then work in the holidays from their own homes. They are very keen on collecting statistics and promoting vaccination programmes.

In the same area local girls are trained as "family-planning counsellors", encouraging the use of the pill, and referring patients to the doctor if there is any problem.[10]

And in Madras, where there is a massive programme to rehouse slum dwellers, young volunteers with secondary education visit families on the new estates, take time to make friends, and then find out tactfully if the children are being immunized and getting extra food, and whether anyone needs medical care. While another young volunteer group from among the residents cleans up the surroundings of the houses and empties the dustbins.

So, contrary to what is sometimes said, there are great resources of able people, especially young ones, willing to give time and energy without payment. But still the most valuable type of volunteer is surely the one who lives on the spot, is the mother of a family and is looked up to by her neighbours.

Joining hands with traditional healers

Next on the ladder come the traditional healers, the village midwives, herbalists, Ayurvedic practitioners and many others, who are found in every community in developing countries.

Although the Chinese Government has recognized the half-million or so traditional practitioners in China, and brought them into the health service to fulfil the "walking on two legs" principle; and the State Government of Tamil Nadu in South India recognizes and encourages Unani and homeopathic doctors—yet in other places the links between traditional and Western-trained health workers are few indeed.

In the Far East middle-aged and respected traditional birth attendants care for 80 to 90% of pregnant women in rural areas. Called "grandmothers", they give support and advice throughout pregnancy, massage the mother during labour, cut the baby's cord and give herbal medicine after delivery to help the uterus to shrink down.

In Thailand many of them have been given a two weeks' course in mother and child care, especially in clean methods of cutting the cord. In Malaysia they have received UNICEF delivery kits; in Indonesia they are trained in maternal and child health clinics.[11]

And at Segbwema in Sierra Leone, where up to 20% of babies get tetanus infection through the cord, 172 traditional midwives have had, with the approval of village chiefs, a one day course in cleanliness during and after labour, and advice on detecting those mothers who are specially at risk. Very brief as this instruction is, it has been effective, with a big drop in the number of babies who suffer from tetanus.[12]

Medical auxiliaries

Now, in what C. H. Wood calls "the continuum of care, knowledge and skill, which stretches from the village mother to the medical specialist", we come to the medical auxiliary.[13]

This is the title given in many countries to the middle-level health worker, the medical assistant, enrolled nurse, assistant nurse-midwife and so on. Usually he or she has had two or three years of post-primary education and then trains for a further two or three years.

Such workers are invaluable. The cost of a medical assistant's training may be only a tenth of that of a doctor's, but he is able to treat 80–90% of the diseases which he will meet in his health centre.

In Malawi all health centres and most hospitals have in recent times been staffed by such auxiliaries. At Port Herald hospital in Malawi, for instance, as Bryant reports, there was no doctor to take charge of the 95 beds, and the principal medical assistant did all the surgery, including Caesarean sections and amputations.[14]

Medical auxiliaries are likely, in contrast to doctors, to be contented with rural life, and to communicate easily with patients who have a traditional outlook.

Giving responsibility to auxiliaries has its problems, however. Professional workers are reluctant to delegate to them.[15] Patients feel they are getting a second-class service. And in some countries the medical assistant grade is trained wholly by Government and so it is difficult for Christian hospitals to obtain their services.

As to a "second-class service", a patient gets looked after much better if a doctor delegates some of his work to a less highly trained person. In Colorado "pediatric nurse practitioners" give almost complete well-child care, and can manage many acute and chronic disorders of children. "Physician's assistants" are trained at Duke University, North Carolina to undertake primary medical care.[16] And in Britain nurses attached to family doctors' partnerships carry out much of the home visiting and are greatly appreciated.

What type of doctor?

What now should be the tasks of those scarce expensive people, doctors and registered nurses, in developing countries?

The answer surely is that they should be team leaders and trainers, spending much of their time teaching and supervising their fellow-workers. As was said earlier, Drs. Raj and Mabelle Arole in Maharastra delegate first-line diagnosis and treatment, including the splinting of fractures, to their nurses, who in turn delegate to assistant nurse-midwives, who train volunteers to give simple drugs.[17]

This runs counter to the Western medical ideal of one-to-one care by doctor for patient. But if the staff is supervised and given constant refresher courses, such team leadership could be the ideal.

A doctor's other chief tasks include investigating and treating the small proportion of patients who have an unusual or very serious illness. And also operating in cases of surgical or obstetric emergency.

Such a picture of what a doctor should do in Third World countries calls for a radical change in methods of health education, in two directions.

Firstly, the medical student must be fully prepared, practically and psychologically, for the work for which he is needed, chief of which is preventive work in a rural setting, where the facilities are limited.

G. L. Monekosso has described the way in which this is to be done in the Cameroons, using a 150 bed "community hospital", with modest facilities. After their initial training in the University, senior students and young doctors will gain experience in the wards of this basic hospital where, as in many mission hospitals, there is no division between medical and surgical patients, and where they become used to very busy outpatient clinics, much emphasis on the care of mothers and children, and simple but adequate laboratory services and equipment.[18]

In China the process has gone much further. At Peking Medical College the course of training for doctors lasts only three years, part of the time being spent in military exercises and gaining physical fitness. After a six-months' period of lectures and demonstrations in medicine, surgery and obstetrics in the medical college, students go with their lecturers to the countryside for nine months practical medical work with a strong preventive bias, as described in chapter 7, before returning to the city for three months of lectures and ward rounds.[19]

The course sounds very short and very basic—even inadequate—compared with the Western curriculum, although in fairness we should remember that the academic year in China lasts for eleven months, so that three academic years in China equal four in the West.[20] Indeed the Chinese agree that the course is still experimental and will need changes.

But to produce doctors who easily adapt to rural life and are able to solve rural health problems is a great achievement indeed.

The other important change needed is that as far as possible all members of the future health team should be trained together, so that they are accustomed to team-work and learn to respect each other's abilities.

This joint training is beginning in Liverpool, where nurses are admitted to the course for the Master in Public Health degree, and attend many of the tropical disease lectures with the doctors.

Again in the Cameroons at Yaoundé, all health professionals and auxiliaries attend the same courses of lectures as far as practicable, and share in team practical work. Some teaching has of course to be given in separate groups. This is a demanding programme, difficult to organize, and for which it is difficult to find teachers. But what promise this integrated flexible approach holds for future medical and allied training.[20]

In Guatemala, too, in spite of opposition from the University, the Government has introduced the combined training of doctors and "rural health technicians", as auxiliaries are called. There is no status difference between the two groups of students, and after qualification they work together in a team in a country where one senior doctor has spoken of his longing to see the integration of health education, farming and labour.[21]

Sometimes it is difficult to believe that such changes as these in medical and nursing education will occur widely, when General Medical Councils and Nursing Councils seem to be as conservative in developing countries as in the West or even more so.

But in fact attitudes to professional education and to the responsibility which different groups should carry are constantly changing. For instance, nurses have recently been trained in Britain to be psychotherapists in mental health units, and the results are very encouraging.[22] Christians have often been prominent in such new types of health training and could be so again.

So should we not hope that in the future Christian medical workers in developing countries will concentrate on training those in the broad lower steps of the pyramid—the mothers, volunteers, traditional midwives and auxiliary nurses? And let us urge that young people who become doctors and registered nurses in State or University Schools should have a training truly relevant to the work for which they are needed, and one which leaves them quite unconcerned about status and prestige.

References Chapter 9

1. De Bono, Edward. *The Use of Lateral Thinking*, Penguin, 1971.
2. Statement at Conference of Ethiopian Medical Association, Addis Ababa, May 1972.
3. *Guardian Weekly*, June 7 1975.
4. Long, E. C. *Tropical Doctor*, April 1972.
5. Lang, Stanley. Report on WHO Conference, Brazzaville, 1974, from Christian Health Association of Nigeria, Lagos.
6. Church, Michael; personal communication.
7. Adey, C. *Saving Health* 1974, **13,** 51.
8. Blumhagen, Rex and Jeanne. Medical Missions' Role in Health Care Delivery (mimeo) MAP, Box 50, Wheaton, Ill.
9. Nickson, P. J. and Fry, S. M.: Final Report of the Medical Assistance Program to the United States Agency for International Development on the Family Planning Grant P10/T 297–110–3–6337003, July 1974.
10. Report of Savar Health Centre, for July 1973–April 1974, Gonoshasthya Kendra PO Nayarhat, District Dacca, Bangladesh.
11. Role of Traditional Birth Attendants in Family Planning, IDRC, Ottawa, 1974.
12. Adey, C. ibid.
13. Wood, C. H. Shortage of Medical Manpower (mimeo) Dar-es-Salaam, 1971.
14. Bryant, J. H. op cit. p. 59.
15. Bryant, J. H. op cit. p. 320.
16. Elliott, Katherine. *Health Manpower and the Medical Auxiliary*, Intermediate Technology Development Group, London, 1971.
17. Mook, Jane Day. AD Magazine of United Church in USA: reprinted in *Vellore Newsletter*, No. 58, March 1974 (36 St George's St, Winchester).
18. Monekosso, G. L. *Tropical Doctor*, 1972, **2,** p. 141.
19. "WHO visits China", *World Health*, September 1974.
20. Nchinda, T. C., *Tropical Doctor*, January 1974, **4,** p. 41.
21. Conference on Medical Auxiliaries and their Value, Oxfam, London, November 30 1974.
22. Marks, I. M., Hallam, R. S., Philpott, R., and Connolly, J. C. *British Medical Journal*, 1975, **3,** pp. 144–148.

Chapter 10

LEARNING TO CO-OPERATE

When brothers work together, mountains are turned into gold. Chinese proverb

In 1966 in the Ankole district of Western Uganda, the death-rate for mothers during pregnancy and labour was 10·74 per 1,000 births, more than fifty times the rate in Britain (see footnote under references.) Keith Masters, a keen young obstetrician, was determined to do something to bring this figure down.

What he did was to call together the leading men in the district, chiefs, teachers and others and explain to them the importance of ante-natal care for all expectant mothers, especially for the "high-risk" ones, for whom labour held special dangers.

He organized extra ante-natal clinics at aid posts—no special buildings needed—and sent mobile medical teams round the country. At the base hospital he had a special "waiting house" for mothers at risk. Lack of transport had been a serious cause of delay in getting mothers to hospital. So dispensaries were each given a big red disc eighteen inches across, and appeals went out over the radio for anyone who saw such a disc by the roadside to give the mother who needed help an urgent lift to hospital. And all midwives were given training in spotting the patient who would need special care.

In four years the maternal death-rate came down to 3·65 deaths for every 1,000 births, and the death rate of babies at the time of birth and immediately afterwards was halved to 67 per 1,000 births.

Of course these figures are still high by European standards, but it was an impressive success, due partly to intensive education at several levels, but also to the practical co-operation achieved.

In the past the hospital had waited for the patient to come, often seeing her arrive in the last stages of exhaustion. Now hospital staff worked actively with community leaders, clinics, midwives and the general public. This team spirit saved many lives.[1]

Linking up in Malawi

The urgent need for church hospitals to co-operate in this way, both with one another, and also with government health services, has been one of the chief tenets of the Christian Medical Commission and its director James McGilvray. The latter has described how such collaboration first started:

"The first of these ventures began in Malawi in 1965. I was in charge of the survey. I well remember the interesting time we had there when, after visiting the Catholic hospital run by the White Sisters, the next port of call was a hospital at Nkhoma operated by the Dutch Reformed Church of South Africa. One of the things that I had seen in this Catholic hospital and which fascinated me very much, was an attempt to train laboratory technicians. And when I looked at the laboratory facilities in the Nkhoma hospital, I could not help but urge the Dutch Reformed doctors to send some of their people for training in the Catholic hospital. After much hesitation the superintendent agreed to accompany me to the Catholic hospital. For the first two minutes or so after he met the Roman Catholic doctor, they were parrying a little, until the Catholic doctor suddenly asked his Reformed colleague what he was doing about certain cases, of which there had recently been a high incidence. Soon they forgot their labels and began talking as men who were dedicated to help those in need. After about an hour, the Dutch Reformed doctor said: 'I would like to send people from Nkhoma Hospital to train here.' And that was a breakthrough. At the end of that survey all the hospitals that had been visited, Catholic, Seventh Day Adventist, Church of God, every one of them, came together to listen to my report. I said: 'The first thing I am going to recommend is that you throw away your labels and come together into one organization.' And they did. When later I showed my report to Dr. Banda, the President, he said: 'This is a miracle. We are very grateful for all the Churches have done in this country, but you'll have noticed that there is no reference to them in our development report for the future. Because,' he said, 'it is impossible to plan with them. Twenty-eight different groups and they haven't yet learned to talk to each other.' I said, 'Well look, sir, now they have agreed to talk to each other and to talk collectively with the Ministry of Health.' And in the most exciting way that organization of Church-related hospitals has come together to work hand in hand with the government, to offer the people new forms of health care.

"They pioneered in all kinds of ways because they've done it selectively and together. They even transfer personnel from one institution to another."[2]

This collaboration between voluntary and Government health workers in Malawi, of which James McGilvray wrote, has led to impressive results in the care of small children.

Dr. Sue Cole-King, a very able pediatrician, was deeply concerned over the plight of children under five in that country. The death rate of children from birth to five years old was 31 to 43%: the corresponding figure in Britain is under 2%. Once again protein-calorie malnutrition was the hidden enemy, weakening resistance to infection.

Dr. Cole-King drew up a plan to provide effective care for 60% of all children in this age group. They were to be seen four times a year, immunized against the common childhood infections, and given tablets to prevent malaria; most important of all, their weight was to be charted regularly and their growth watched carefully. Their mothers were to be taught the simple principles of health.

Church medical workers and Peace Corps volunteers co-operated with Government, seminars were held to train medical auxiliaries, and the early results were most encouraging. 30% of Malawi's children under the age of five were enrolled in child health clinics in the first two years, and the proportion of those who were underweight dropped from 37% to 28% during this period. One of the factors in this success, remarks Susan Cole-King, was the joint recognition by different bodies of the importance of the scheme.[3]

Fighting tuberculosis on the North-west Frontier

In many parts of the world similar experiments in co-operation are being tried with great benefit. In Pakistan two women doctors, Dr. Pfau and Dr. Gogel, have been working for the Damien Foundation on the control of leprosy. They were encouraged by Government to set up field clinics and train young men as "leprosy technicians".

They found that parts of Pakistan are almost free from leprosy, and so Dr. Gogel has been concentrating on the North West Frontier Province where more leprosy patients are to be found, and has set up clinics in remote areas such as Swat.

The technicians, who are Government employees, are very much on their own, and make long journeys with much hill climbing in order to reach distant villages. The Damien Foundation supplies the drugs and supervises their work. But the two doctors realized that some of the clinics have only a small register of patients, and they thought "Why shouldn't we add tuberculosis control to our programme?"

TB is perhaps the biggest single disease problem (if one excludes malnutrition) in Pakistan today. There are reckoned to be two million sufferers from it, or almost one in every twenty of the population. And effective treatment, which requires careful supervision for at least two years in most cases, is virtually impossible because of the difficulty in follow-up.

Dr. Gogel was a little embarrassed when she explained their methods to me. "We don't use X-rays" she pointed out, "and we don't usually give streptomycin injections either." "That's fine," I replied. I had read the Oxfam memo on TB control in developing countries, and it is their policy, which Pakistan endorses, to keep everything as simple as possible.

So TB is diagnosed by testing the sputum for tubercle bacilli, easily done in rural conditions, and treated by tablets of isoniazid and thiacetazone combined, which the technicians issue. The great secret is following up the patients and making sure that they take their tablets. This can never be done from hospitals, but the technicians achieve it. In addition, all the children who can be reached are inoculated with BCG so that the next generation is protected. And Government doctors give a varying amount of supervision.

This Damien Foundation scheme, the most impressive attack on TB which I found in Pakistan, was a most effective form of co-operation between a voluntary body (non-missionary in this instance) and the national Government, and produced far-reaching benefits.

Looking to the future

Hakan Hellberg, writing in 1971 on the future of church-related work in Africa where Protestant, Anglican and Orthodox Churches had 645 medical institutions and the Catholic Church probably a similar number, stressed the importance of such joint action.

He foresaw a period of ten to twenty years of difficult transition from church-related to Government-directed health care. This, he believed, would take place at different speeds in different countries. The churches would come to concentrate on providing *people* for different levels of medical care, and would be less and less involved in the ownership of institutions.

Christian doctors and nurses would sometimes be employed by Government, sometimes by the churches, and sometimes by a mixture of both.

In this transition period much consultation would be needed. Western agencies would have to discuss the future with African leaders. Church must consult with church, and the churches jointly with Government. Seminars would be needed to draw up plans for coming days, and to select areas of work for special study.

In short, he foresaw a great need for a continuous process of re-education, sharing of information, and joint planning.[4]

This process is in fact already going on, but requires to be intensified. Every established undertaking in Christian health care should be reviewing its links with other Christian enterprises, its relationships with the Government, and its place in the whole pattern of health provision, to see if it can co-operate with others more fruitfully than ever.

References **Chapter 10**

1. Masters, K. W. *Maternity Services in Ankole* (mimeo).
2. McGilvray, J. C. *Missionalia*, April 3 1975, Pretoria.
3. Cole-King, Sue. *Some thoughts on meeting MCH Needs in Malawi*, February 1972 (mimeo). Present address: Institute of Development Studies, University of Sussex.
4. Hellberg, J. H. *Church-related Medical Work in Africa*, February 1971, Christian Medical Commission, Geneva.

Footnote to page 62

The comparison is not exact, because the Ankole figure is for mothers who delivered in hospital and rural units only, and the British figure is for the entire population. The death-rate of *all* mothers in Ankole, which is not known, would probably be lower. But the contrast in rates would still be very great.

Chapter 11

UNSUSPECTED HUMAN RICHES

In a special unit in Barlinnie prison, Glasgow, are five men serving life sentences. Four are murderers. Three years ago one of them was in solitary confinement in the segregation unit in Inverness prison, the grimly-named "cage". The others all have records as "hard men".

Today they are learning sculpture and the guitar, making toys, and one is training as a chef. They are on Christian-name terms with the staff. Decisions about work and activities are community decisions, made by prisoners and staff after joint discussion.

The sculptor, who has qualified for the Open University after three years study, so as to read for a degree in Sociology, says "They treat you like a human being here. Before, I was living in a jungle."

Described as an "impressive exercise in community relations", and owing much to the devotion of the staff, all of whom have volunteered for the task, this whole experiment highlights the remarkable degree to which unsuspected human resources will flower in a climate of understanding and encouragement.[1]

Latent resources in old age

Dr. Brian Lodge, consultant psychiatrist at Carlton Hayes Hospital in Leicestershire, is another great believer in this approach. He looks after many elderly patients who are labelled as suffering from "senile dementia", a label which he dislikes and ignores. He believes that such patients have many capabilities only waiting to be drawn out.

So he asked Frank Parker, headmaster of Craven Lodge School, Melton Mowbray, to see what he could do. Six women patients were chosen, suffering from moderately severe senile dementia. Their memories were very poor; they were confused about where they were and what time of year it was; they were apathetic and incontinent, and according to the statistics, one of them would die within six months.

The aim of the teacher was to make their lives richer and happier by recreating personal identity, redeveloping personal responsibility and encouraging them to remember past events.

How was this achieved? The nurses were encouraged to talk to the patients all the time. Patients had newspapers or magazines read to them, discussed the events described, and recalled similar happenings from their own experience in past years. Simple indoor gardening was taken up, as well as ward cooking and the laying of tables for meals.

Letters were written, games played, social afternoons and flower picking expeditions arranged, and all the time there was talking and talking.

Every small task was a chance for discussion and encouragement. What shall we put in the cake, what are the steps in making it, how long should it be baked for? The staff were to create opportunities for praise and leave room for initiative.

The teaching staff insisted that the room should be brightened up. Full-length mirrors were provided as well as large clocks, calendars, pictures and places for personal possessions.

The patients chose their clothes, chose the menu, set the table, helped with the cooking, and were consulted about their personal appearance.

What were the results? Within eight weeks the old ladies, previously bedridden, were moving about the ward, and all incontinence had stopped. After ten weeks they had settled in to the new occupations. At the end of six months no one had died, and standards of dressing, food preparation, social intercourse and independence were all reported as "very satisfactory".

Frank Parker concluded "Now I look with seeing eyes on old age."[2]

L'Arche

This same urge to develop the rich human potential of those whom society rejects has been pre-eminently felt by Jean Vanier, founder of L'Arche (the Ark), a community for the mentally handicapped.

Jean, the son of General Vanier, a distinguished soldier, was a naval cadet in Britain and later a naval officer on Canada's only aircraft-carrier. In his cadet days a report was sent to the General that Jean lacked respect for his senior officers. "As long as he never shows a lack of respect for those under him, he'll be all right", the General responded happily, as Bill Clarke records. Such respect has been one of the key-notes of L'Arche.

Jean soon left the Navy to search for a community where he could live the Gospel in a spirit of poverty. After various experiments, he settled in Trosly, a village in the forest of Compiègne, in France; he chose a house, L'Arche, near Val Fleuri, a home for mentally handicapped young men.

Into his house he took Raphael and Philippe, men who had had long experience as patients in big mental hospitals. His aim was to live with such men, long rejected by society and made to feel worthless, and show them love and acceptance as people.

Since 1964 Vanier's community has spread all over the village, and similar communities have been founded in England, North America and Bangalore in India. In each place mentally handicapped men and women share the life of a family with the "assistants", many of them volunteers—all working, playing, singing, sharing meals and worshipping together.

Vanier's original aim was to welcome the rejects of society with kindness and compassion. But soon he noticed the gifts and potential of handicapped people. Philippe had made a collection of slides to entertain his friends. Raphael saved matches and chocolates to give to children in the village. They could indeed give to others. Vanier realized that "if the handicapped are sustained by loving relationships, they are capable of progressing in an astonishing way."

The spirit of L'Arche is one of warm acceptance and appreciation of each man and woman, and deep respect for their personality—a respect which is one of L'Arche's most enriching attributes.

In this atmosphere those who come to help learn much from the men at L'Arche; their simplicity of spirit, their affection and readiness to welcome others, their generosity and unquestioning faith call out a response from the others, allowing them to be simpler and more truly themselves in their turn. Vanier saw that the handicapped, with their gifts of the heart, could do as much or more for society as society could do for them.

The life of each community is sustained by worship together, where, particularly in the Holy Communion, the distinction between the handicapped and the assistants totally disappears, and each person appears, as Bill Clarke so aptly says, "as a child of God, redeemed by the death and resurrection of Jesus." In this fellowship André can say to Claude, "You know, Claude, Jesus calms your nerves", and all can share in choruses of "Alleluias".[3]

Warmth of friendship

What emerges from many of the modern experiments in caring for the handicapped or rejected is not only the way in which human resources are allowed to develop, but the extent to which ordinary people, without any special professional qualifications, play an essential part in such flowering of personality.

This is well illustrated at Honeylands Hospital, Exeter, which has been since 1967 a "family support unit" for mentally and physically handicapped children with severe and often multiple handicaps.

The atmosphere in the hospital is informal, with nurses and therapists wearing slacks instead of uniform, and play-group leader and volunteers taking an active part alongside the consultants and registrars from the Royal Devon and Exeter Hospital. The aim is to reproduce the quality of an extended family, in which each member has his own particular talents and particular difficulties.

Mothers feel supported, knowing that they can discuss their problems over and over again with the staff, and that when the stage has been reached at which a child can be cared for at home, the hospital will always take him back again to give his mother a weekend break.

Churches and the Red Cross arrange holiday trips. University students and sixth-formers organize swimming and pony-riding, and children of volunteers come to the hospital to play games, and join in beach activities, together with scouts and guides. Friendships made between handicapped children and volunteers persist well after the children have left Honeylands.[4]

There seem to be so many similar experiments—but still not nearly enough—in linking mental patients, in particular, with the community at large.

At Brentry Hospital for the Subnormal near Bristol there is an Aunt and Uncle Group, formed by men and women aged 50 to 60, who develop a one-to-one relationship with "high-grade" patients and take them out. A Youth Club organizes play therapy for the "low-grade" patients. Brunel Technical College students have built an adventure playground with a tower slide, and platforms in trees.[5]

The Accepting Community

And at Aro, in Nigeria, encouraged by Dr. Lambo, a psychiatrist of international reputation, four villages have formed a therapeutic community.

Psychiatric patients attend the day hospital in the central village, returning late in the evening to the homes nearby where they are fed and housed.

In this way they keep in touch all the time with a social environment that is familiar and reassuring. The village community is tolerant and sympathetic, and friendly intercourse is easy and free.

Patients are accompanied by their relatives, and all of them attend social and church activities in the usual way. For those who need long-term care and supervision, work is found on neighbouring farms.[6]

All this is nothing new in European experience, as Lambo says. At Geel in Belgium, the community has welcomed psychiatric patients for hundreds of years.

They were brought to Geel's Church of St. Dympna in the Middle Ages, and after a period in the "sickroom", managed by a college of canons, they lived with families in houses surrounding the church.

In spite of ups and downs through the centuries, the tradition of family care has been maintained ever since.

Today patients come to the State Psychiatric Hospital for a period of preliminary observation and assessment. Then all who are not too handicapped are placed in families. The family receives an allowance for the care they provide, varying from 110 Fr. (£1 40, $3) a day upwards, according to the accommodation provided and the patient's needs. Each patient has his own room, and shares meals, recreation, household chores and social life in general with the family.

Formerly most families were farmers, and so he would help on the farm. Today he may give a hand in running the family business, or do odd jobs. If he cannot find full-time work, he will join the pre-industrial training programme in the hospital workshop.

The foster family appreciates his contribution and treats him like its own relative.

He is free to take part in the life of the town just like anyone else, watching the Sunday Soccer game and going to the cinema.

He may join in fishing competitions and contribute to the annual art exhibition.

As Dr. Matheussen, head of the psychiatric hospital, points out, Geel provides a "tolerant environment of non-specifically trained citizens" which is so valuable.

Patients feel accepted and emotionally supported by their foster families. Instead of the dependency and passivity which an institution produces they gain independence and freedom in the town's open community, and achieve a "positive self-image", as the phrase goes.

Geel, explains Dr. Matheussen, is not some kind of "reservation" or "colony" for mental patients. It is just like any other Belgian community, modern, and sharing in the changes which are affecting all Europe. It has just one difference. The culturally conditioned deep-seated fear of the mentally ill does not exist there.[7]

In all these accounts of the interplay of human relationships a certain pattern can be seen emerging.

Groups of individuals, whether hard-core prisoners, mentally handicapped men or elderly women, are seen as persons of great worth with rich inner resources waiting to be drawn out and shared with others.

As they meet with appreciation, acceptance and respect for their personalities, so they respond in many-facetted ways. Where possible they move out from the institution into the community, becoming a part of it, profiting from the care and concern of those around them, but also contributing a great deal of love, warmth and simplicity.

And impressively enough, those who play a major part in this recovery of becoming truly human do not need to have professional skills. The experts are there, in the background. But the closest contact, the most meaningful relationship, comes from the ordinary friend or neighbour, volunteer or student. In this way every Christian is able to serve his fellows in widely varying styles of "long-term loving", and gains great rewards as he does so.

References **Chapter 11**

1. *The Guardian*, July 25 1974.
2. *Times Educational Supplement*, August 9 1974.
3. Clarke, Bill. *Enough Room for Joy*, Darton, Longman & Todd, London, 1974.
4. Brimblecombe, F. S. W. *British Medical Journal*, 1974, **4,** p. 706.
5. *The Guardian*, May 22 1974.
6. Lambo, Prof Adeoye. "The Village of Aro", Ch. 20 in *Medical Care in Developing Countries*, by Maurice King, Oxford, 1966.
7. The State Psychiatric Hospital, Centre for Family Care, Geel, 1975.

Chapter 12

WITH HEALING IN HIS WINGS

"Go to the witch doctor," they said to Simon Mundeta. "He'll find out who caused your illness and why. The doctors here can't do much more for you." "No, no," he flung back, "I can't do it. It's better to die here on my bed than go back to that." So his friends prayed and sang hymns, he was given supportive treatment, and slowly he recovered from his severe and longstanding kidney infection.

F. Donaldson tells the story of Mr. Mundeta in his account of the experimental study which was carried out in the Sister Buck Memorial Hospital at Chikore, Rhodesia.[1]

For years the staff had been feeling that Western medicine was not fully adequate. The traditional religion of the Shona people did not make any separation between healing and religion. But orthodox Christianity appeared to insist on a wide distinction, and so church members would go off to the other sects which emphasized healing.

Many observers have emphasized that a patient in Africa wants to know "Why?"—"Why did it happen to me?" Listen to Una Maclean of Nigeria: "A palm-wine tapper whose rope snaps as he is suspended high above the ground, and who fractures his femur, is perfectly aware that the frayed rope was involved in his misfortune. But this will not prevent his wondering why it should have happened to him in particular on that very day, up that particular palm tree. The demonstration that his rope must have been in a decrepit condition will not satisfy his search for the real, underlying cause of his accident."[2]

Indeed the question is truly not Why? but *Who?* Who has done this thing to me? "The influences which proceed directly from one individual to another," continues Una Maclean, "are of the greatest importance in Yoruba thought, and the key to the understanding of Nigerian medicine."

At Chikore the staff realized that if these questions went unanswered, patients would not feel themselves cured. Something more than Western medicine was needed.

So among the trees in the grounds of this 36-bedded hospital they built a round hut, thatched like a chief's house; it was *gome ra Jehovah*, the house of the Lord. It was a place in which all Africans felt at home.

The Rev. Simon Mundeta was aged 50 at that time, a true pastor, quiet, trusted, radiating an impression of goodwill and integrity. He was deeply interested in spiritual healing and his long illness had given him a keen sympathy for other sufferers.

As in other parts of Africa, the traditional religion of the patients centred on their ancestors, with whom they formed, as Jansen[3] says, one solid family group. The ancestors can easily be slighted or displeased and then punish their descendants. In addition there are the "Royal Spirits", the gods who once were men, and also the lesser spirits of trees and waterfalls, all capable of causing illness and disaster.

Mr. Mundeta was left free to make his own plans. He would visit the wards, hold services and sit by a patient's bedside. But mostly he spent his time in the *gome*. A patient would quietly come to him for a talk and they would sit together by the fire—Mrs. Mundeta joining them when the patient was a woman.

The pastor would listen while the patient talked. Then they would discuss together. Mr. Mundeta maintains that the spirits are there, just as the New Testament describes them; but the Holy Spirit when in our lives is stronger than any other spirit, and Jesus can take away all fear, and heal every situation. All this he would share with the patient.

They would go on talking, praying and singing hymns together.

Donaldson believes that in this small friendly hospital, where children often romp and play, Western medicine and spiritual counselling reinforce each other, producing an enhanced total effect. While the patient's malaria and hookworm anaemia is being treated, his long-standing fears can be resolved and family quarrels healed.

Western medicine, asserts Donaldson, is too materialistic and limited. African culture covers the whole of life, no doubt seeing events too personally or too much in the form of influence by spirits, but still presenting a world-view which includes all life.

Scientific medicine needs other ways of healing to supplement it, healing through frank discussion of problems, through reconciliation, through prayer and active faith.

It is an attractive picture—the small welcoming hospital where children are free to run about, the wise understanding pastor with his confidence that "victory is to the Lord", and the mutual trust between pastor and doctor, from which the patient benefits.

The whole account raises two questions—What should be the relation between scientific and "spiritual" healing, and how can a traditional world view be reconciled with a Christian scientific approach to life?

The two questions are really intertwined but it may be easier to try and separate them, dealing with the second one in another chapter.

Jesus saves

The basic message of Christianity, say Francis MacNutt, is that Jesus saves.[4] He saves from sin, ignorance, weakness of purpose and physical sickness. He brings new life.

To prove the genuineness of his ministry, Jesus declared that "the lame walk, lepers are cleansed and the deaf hear, and the poor have good news preached to them."[5] The cures were good news in action, part of the message that Jesus sets men free.

He sent his disciples out to cure diseases and heal the sick.[6] When Peter in *Acts* wants to describe Jesus in a few words, he speaks of Him as doing good and curing all who had fallen into the power of the devil.[7] And Peter himself, with Philip and others, demonstrated Christ's power to heal, in the early days of the Church.[8]

Sometimes it seemed, as Dick Lyth has said, that Jesus wasn't sure which to do first, whether to cure the illness or forgive the sin.[9] And *St. James*, at the end of his epistle, mentions both these great happinesses in the same breath.[10] Men and women are whole people, body and spirit cannot be completely separated, and each person needs the help of God who is his Creator as well as his Redeemer.

Claiming the healing of love

And He is not only that, goes on MacNutt. He is a loving Father, generous and compassionate. Why should we think of Him as disapproving and critical, instead of enjoying with him a warm Father-Son relationship? "How much more does your Father in heaven give good things . . ." (*St. Matthew* 7.11) We should expect that God wishes to heal.[11]

Such healing is specially needed by those who have been hurt in childhood, perhaps in the first years of life. Maybe they felt rejected or unloved by their parents. How often these effects seem to go on and on from one generation to the next, with the unloved child becoming the withdrawn undemonstrative young parent, unable in her turn to give the love her child needs.

This gives an opportunity for her friends to ask that Jesus should heal these wounds, with His love filling the empty places in the heart, or that the love of a Heavenly Father should more than make up for the lack of a human parent's love.[12]

The ministry of counselling

The growth of Christian counselling has provided a wonderful development in healing at the present time. Joyce Peel, a CMS missionary in S. India, has written: "My introduction to counselling came through research in writing a play on the problem of suicide. I contacted Dr. Sarada Menon, the psychiatrist at the Government mental hospital here, and she directed me to meet patients at the general hospital. I went there with the Rev. Mahimai Rufus, one of our clergy, who was trained in counselling at Vellore. We were given a doctor's consulting room and a boy was brought to us. He had attempted suicide, but all he could tell the doctors was that it was due to stomach and headache. I watched to see how Mr. Rufus dealt with him, and how, by the way in which he listened—it took at least half an hour—the boy finally came out with the real story; a love affair and family quarrel. I then offered to visit an Anglo-Indian lady and the hospital gave me her address. I had two long interviews with her, one at her home and one in mine, and I found that she got great relief just by pouring out her troubles and knowing she had a friend outside the family where her troubles were. I could also give back to her the facts she gave me in some sort of order that gave her new insights—something Mr. Rufus had taught me.

"Dr. Sarada was very pleased about all this. The doctors simply do not have time to listen for hours to patients who have attempted suicide—about three a day at the general hospital—and a welcome awaits us at the hospital, and an encouragement to do as much work in this direction as we have time for."[13]

Praying for physical healing

But when it comes to praying for the healing of physical disease by spiritual means many Christian doctors have reservations. They feel that this might lead to the neglect of necessary treatment of a scientifically-based kind.

Arnold Aldis, a distinguished Christian surgeon, urges that while God is the source of all healing, He normally supplies it through the means He has provided, that is through the skill of doctors and nurses. The miracles of New Testament times were to authenticate God's message at certain critical periods. As God normally feeds mankind through the farmer's sowing and harvest, so He normally heals through the applied knowledge of men and through natural means.[14]

But, extremely important as modern medical care is, God's healing power cannot be limited to this channel only. So often when His Spirit is bringing new life to men and women, there is a spring-time for the body as well as the soul, and physical health blossoms and grows with the changed personality.

And there is a growing realization that at times of illness we need not only the skilled help which is so essential, but the love and support of friends, their care in the days of recovery, and above all God's love and power at work throughout the illness. Indeed Aldis stresses this, reminding us that prayer and faith are vitally important and that often we under-estimate the place of prayer in the healing process.

It was the team-work in the Sister Buck hospital at Chikore that was the secret of success. And this should be the pattern, doctor and pastor working closely together to help their patients. Doctors, says MacNutt, should pray for their patients that God will do what they cannot do, or do what they can do but do it better and faster and more cheaply! Doctors, counsellors and other church members can claim God's grace together.

Prayer and the village fellowship

But perhaps the picture at Chikore is not altogether the ideal one. We need a model of healing by varied means which does not depend on a hospital or a doctor or even on a gifted pastor. In developing countries hospitals, doctors and pastors are all very scarce. Just as ordinary day-to-day medical care in many places must be given by the village health worker and the volunteer, so must prayer for healing, in faith and love, be the duty of the ordinary Christian fellowship in the village. The two types of service would reinforce each other.

Christians would thus show their concern for the whole of man's personality, and witness to the power of the one who came "with healing in His wings".[15]

Lessons from independent Churches

Can we learn something of how to do this from the independent churches in Africa? Some of these were founded largely because, as Mitchell[16] says, "the mission churches did not consider the possibility of providing a context for healing which would offer a spiritual power for the commonly-believed-in spiritual causes of illness."

In traditional Yoruba thinking, sickness and health affect the whole of a man's personality, physical and psychological, his relationships with other men and women, and also with non-human forces and entities.[17]

But in the past, the older Christian churches had seemed too "other-worldly", with Christianity insufficiently related to African life. And so these new churches had sprung up.

As an example, the Ijebu Ode group was born in Nigeria as an Anglican prayer group, during the influenza pandemic of 1918. Neither Western medicine nor the Anglican church itself seemed able to offer any protection against this virulent disease. And the group did not want to turn to traditional medicine. So it rejected both modern and Yoruba medicine in favour of faith in Jesus Christ and fervent prayer, and the members went forward encouraged by a small American faith-healing group called Faith Tabernacle.

This was the beginning of the Aladura churches, "Aladura" meaning "praying man". These churches have varied titles and emphases, the older ones in particular having many of the ordinary activities of the mission-founded churches, such as worship services, schools and church societies. But healing activity is their greatest attraction and attribute.

The ministers are prophets who act as both pastors and healing practitioners, being the Christian counterparts of the diviner-healer of traditional medicine.

Many people come to the prophet as a man who has power with God, and ask to be cured of sickness, or often in the case of women, infertility; to be protected against witchcraft, or to be granted success in life.

The prophet will pray over the patient and receive a "vision" from God, telling him the cause of the patient's trouble, and the treatment needed. The cause may be some natural factor, or witchcraft, or personal sin.

The treatment is by vigorous prayer, either in church or in the prophet's house, by holy water for washing or drinking, and by holy oil, rubbed on or taken as a draught.

Hermione Harris[17] has described the life of the Cherubim and Seraphim church in London, a branch of one of the leading Aladura groups. It attracts many Nigerian students and their wives, the men anxious for success in exams, the women concerned to have children and to be preserved from danger in childbirth. Difficulties of accommodation in the city, trouble with the police, and worry over the family at home in Africa are all brought to the prophet. And central in the minds of many is the need to be protected against misfortune, whether examination failure, mental breakdown, or outside enemies.

The Cherubim and Seraphim church deals with these practical problems of life in much the same way as traditional religion has done, and this is the great attraction.

What are the lessons which these churches teach? Certainly we should pray for each other's practical needs, particularly for health and recovery from illness, especially remembering the element of anxiety and stress which enters into nearly every episode of sickness. We should be concerned about each other's work, studies, family and home and bring these to God. And personal relationships are vitally important too. All these should mean much to a caring fellowship.

But wealth and success in life are not the goals of Christian living. Health is important, but a right relationship with God is more important still. How can we get a balanced approach?

Simon Barrington-Ward[18] declares that the Aladura movement, among similar cults, was never able adequately to bring its private religious resources to bear on the public world, the political and economic world. He calls for something that will be a pattern for the *whole* of life, inspiring our technological, complex and pluriform society.

Bengt Sundkler[19] said of the Zionist churches in South Africa that their marked emphasis on healing and their warm congregational support could not bring sufferers out of the vicious circle of malnutrition, low wages and low social status.

Do we need Christian congregations which are deeply concerned to pray for sick friends and neighbours, perhaps in small informal groups which include their relatives, with a strong reliance on Christ's victorious power over adverse spiritual and psychological forces? And if so, will the same congregations be equally concerned for the success of the technical medical skills and social and political efforts which are also needed so that healing may be complete? We greatly need more light on this problem.

Chapter 12

1. Donaldson, F. *The Sister Buck Memorial Hospital Project, Chikore, Rhodesia.* Christian Medical Commission, Geneva (mimeo) 1966–1967.
2. Maclean, Una. *Magical Medicine,* Penguin, London, 1971.
3. Jansen, G. *The Doctor-Patient Relationship in an African Tribal Society*, Van Gorcum and Co. BV, Assen, The Netherlands, 1973, p. 29.
4. MacNutt, Francis, *Healing,* Ave Maria Press, Notre Dame, Indiana, 1974, p. 49.
5. *St. Matthew* 11. 5.
6. *St. Luke* 9. 1–2.
7. *Acts* 10. 38.
8. *Acts* 3. 6–7, 8. 5–8.
9. Lyth, R. *Mission to the Under-loved,* Ruanda Mission, CMS, London.
10. *St. James* 5. 14–15.
11. MacNutt F. p. 100.
12. ibid. pp. 183–6.
13. Peel, Joyce. Link Letter, Sept. 17 1973, CMS, London.
14. Aldis, Arnold. "Biblical Teaching on Healing", *Inter Medicos*, **1,** 1975, 18 arg. Rikshospitalet, Oslo, p. 27.
15 *Malachi* 4.2. AV.
16. Mitchell, Robert C. *Witchcraft, Sin, Divine Power and Healing*, Christian Medical Commission, Geneva, 1968.
17. Harris, Hermione. "The Cherubim and Seraphim Church", Seminar on Christianity in Post-Colonial Africa, May 9 1974, School of Oriental and African Studies, London.
18. Barrington-Ward, S. "The Centre Cannot Hold; Spirit Possession as Redefinition". Seminar on Christianity in Post-Colonial Africa, May 2 1974, SOAS, London.
19. Sundkler, Bengt G. M. *Bantu Prophets in South Africa*, Oxford University Press, London, 1961.

Chapter 13

WEB OF LIFE

"One day Monda was very ill, cold and clammy, and Wilaki, the traditional healer, explained that she had insulted her husband Kauyu. So the spirit of her mother-in-law had taken away part of Monda's spirit.

"Wilaki took out seven pieces of wood which angry ancestors had shot into Monda's body. Kauyu, who goes regularly to church, told Monda to confess her fault and promise to do better. He prayed to God for his wife, asked the ancestors to put back her spirit, rubbed her with leaves and blew on her body. She soon recovered."

Donald McGregor comments on this case-history from Papua, New Guinea, that although the illness may have been malaria, there was a problem of behaviour and relationships which had upset the balance which should exist in the larger family of ancestors and living men.

The world view of Monda and Kauyu, in which spiritual beings inter-penetrated their everyday life, supported an ethical system which censured anger, laziness, and stealing and held the family together. It enabled a community to live together, perhaps for centuries, and seen from within it appeared wholly logical and consistent.[1]

Jansen, a Dutch missionary doctor working in the Transkei, insists that a doctor should study and understand all that he can of the cultural values of the people among whom he works. Then he will be able to bridge the gap between his own outlook, which is inclined to be too materialistic and technological, and that of his patient who sees events in terms of personal causes and spirit influences.

This inter-cultural barrier, often very great even between people who belong to the same nation but differ in education and social customs, has to be overcome if the patients' attitudes to illness are to be sympathetically understood.[2]

"Overcoming the barrier" really means doctor (or nurse) and patient being able to understand each other, and sharing as far as possible the same concepts—not only the same words, but the same meaning of the words.

This is far from easy, especially in health education, where it may be difficult for a parent to see the need to protect a child against an illness which is only a possibility in the distant future. Therefore much insight and mutual trust is called for, if preventive health measures—which may bring hard work and inconvenience to many people—are likely to succeed.

So the Christian health worker from overseas—or even from the nearby city—must understand cultural beliefs. But the difficulty is that these are always changing.

"Culture, whether African, British, or Red Indian is not static. It evolves, it changes", says a Nigerian writer.[3] And Dr Bolaji Idowu speaks of a religious vacuum appearing in Africa today.

"The keynote of the Yoruba's life", he explains, "is religion. It forms the foundation and all-governing principle of life for him. The religious cult includes shrines, a priesthood, a highly developed system of sacrifice, and festivals of music, dancing, singing and drama. Alongside this is a moral code, including chastity, hospitality, generosity, truth, rectitude, honesty, protection of women, family solidarity, and respect for elders.

"Today there exists nearly a religious vacuum: much of the old pagan religion has gone for many urban or near-urban Yorubas."[4]

But if there is indeed a disappearance of much of the old fabric of life, with all that this implies, belief in traditional medicine still exists. 72% of families in Old Ibadan in Nigeria in the early 1960's used traditional medicines "sometimes" or "always".[5]

What can western-trained medical workers learn from traditional healers, and how is a whole system of magico-religious care for sickness to be assessed in Christian terms?

Here the advice and help of national Christian leaders is essential. "The problem of deciding what is Christian or unChristian in African culture is still with us today . . . the proper attitude would be to revive whatever is good and compatible with Christianity", says an African writer.[6]

One lesson from traditional medicine—the putting of a concern for healing fully into the framework of religious belief and practice—has been discussed in a previous chapter. I would like to look at three other areas where there is so much to be learnt.

Support at times of crisis

Firstly, special support is given at important crises in life. Childbirth is one example, and as Una Maclean says, "for women everywhere, even with modern care, pregnancy and labour are a period of relative hazard."[7]

So in Accra most pregnant women still flock to the traditional midwife for protective medicine, even though they use modern maternity services. Educated and uneducated alike need the security of the protective waist belt.

And in the valley of the Ica, Peru, the local midwives or *parteras* are popular because they understand the mothers' beliefs about the "hot" and "cold" properties of different medicines, and the mothers find group solidarity and support within their home surroundings.

Recovery from serious illness is another deeply important event. When a Nigerian mental patient has recovered in the home of a *babalawo* or diviner, he goes in the simple garment which he wore during his illness down to the river-side.

There a dove is sacrificed over his head. The sacrificial blood is used to wash him and then the dead dove and his garment are cast down stream, while the priest recites verses which end . . .

> As the river can never flow backwards
> So may this illness never return.

After this vivid ceremony, so strikingly reminiscent of the Old Testament rite of "cleansing the leper" with the sacrifice of a bird over running water, as portrayed in *Leviticus* 14, the patient returns to a feast with his waiting relatives. The stigma of his illness has been completely blotted out, and he is fully restored to society.[8]

Could pregnancy and labour be times when patients are especially assured, in church-related clinics, of God's fatherly love and power to protect? And could the time of discharge from hospital after serious illness be made an opportunity for a brief time of praise in which the relatives could join?

Insight into the causes of anxiety

The second area is that of simple psychotherapy. The traditional practitioners of China provide valuable emotional support to their patients, spending long hours in caring for them.[9] The *babalawo* of Ibadan, diviner-priests, are skilled psychotherapists and willing to care for frank psychoses too. T. A. Lambo, the psychiatrist, asks them to help their modern counterparts in the Aro village settlement by assessing patients and even helping with their treatment.[10]

As Christians we surely need the same concern for those who are anxious, depressed or confused, and the same solicitude for them as persons, with similar insight into family problems and the social factors of the illness. Perhaps the skilled Christian counsellor will fill this gap in our health care, and give the support and understanding that so many people need.

Can herbal medicines help?

And lastly, is there no place for herbal medicines in Christian health care? We western doctors must frankly acknowledge that many patients whom we see do not need active modern drugs at all.

James Mackenzie, the famous general practitioner turned heart specialist who died about fifty years ago, laid it down that "in half the cases a doctor sees in (general) practice he is unable to . . . make a rational diagnosis." The symptoms are vague and ill-defined and on physical examination nothing abnormal can be found.[11] This still holds true today. K. B. Thomas, a doctor in Portsmouth, could not make a firm diagnosis in 43% of the patients who consulted him, and the great majority of them got better without any active treatment.[12]

If this is true in other countries too, and my general impression would confirm its truth in Africa, what is the value of treating such patients with imported drugs which only act as placebos? Ideally no drug treatment at all need be given, but if this is too much to insist on, why not give herbal medicine which is cheap and trusted because it is familiar, so long as it is proved to be harmless?

Such restraint in the use of modern remedies would go some way to meet Illich's strictures that western drugs are often used ineffectively, and may be damaging in their side-effects.[13] The same can be said of herbal medicines of course, but I incline to think that modern drugs, when not used with considerable skill and care, have the greater power to cause harm.

If we condemn traditional medicines entirely, what is to happen to the vast rural areas of the world where there is one doctor to fifty thousand people or more, and, as in parts of India, the family may only have 5p ($0.10) a day to spend on all their needs?[14]

The chief difficulty for Christians is that these remedies are part of a magico-religious philosophy in which the plant preparations are only really effective if the power of the gods are invoked by incantations.

Mitchell has said that Yoruba drugs of proved therapeutic value are "inextricably set in a matrix of sacrifice, prayer and magic in such a way that recourse to Yoruba medicine was a resort to Yoruba religion or, in the eyes of Christian Yoruba, paganism."[15]

Some medicines are frankly charms, applied for instance to a ring which then gives the wearer special influence over others. The link with witchcraft is puzzling but real. Traditional doctors may protect their patients against the effects of witchcraft, but at the same time they say "We depend on them (witches). They are the mothers."[16]

However, every culture has its household remedies for mild complaints, and practises self-medication, whether in Ibadan or London.

And magic is not needed where common sense would do. Jansen quotes Malinowski as saying of the Melanesians "in the lagoon fishing where man can rely completely upon his knowledge and skill, magic does not exist, while in the open-sea fishing, full of danger and uncertainty, there is extensive magical ritual to secure safety and good results."[17] For well-known conditions common-sense treatment is all that is needed, and in Zulu culture what is considered as "natural" illness is treated by herbal (or natural) medicines.[18]

So there does appear to be a range of folk-medicine, even if limited, which is not bound up with magic, and so scope exists for a fresh look at herbal treatment.

The early independent African churches in Lagos in the 1890's were deeply interested in providing such simple medical care. They experimented with "Christian native medicine", some of the Church leaders being practising herbalists, and separated the curative properties of traditional herbs from their associated rites and sacrifices. Unfortunately this excellent experiment never became widely adopted by their churches, and dropped out of view.[19]

There is a second difficulty, however, that of assessing accurately the potency and value of different herbal preparations. Research in this field went on in Kampala for some years. But each plant may contain many alkaloids, all of which have to be tested for effectiveness; the potency differs in the fresh and the dried plant; the amount of rainfall alters the strength of the potent principle in the herbs; and dosage is so vague—no fixed quantity being used—that it is very hard to make a meaningful assay.

Nevertheless if at least some herbal medicines could be listed which would relieve symptoms without being toxic, and if Christian leaders in the countries concerned could accept them as free from magical associations, then "whatever is good and compatible with Christianity" in traditional medicine could indeed be known and widely used.

References Chapter 13

1. McGregor, Donald. "Traditional Beliefs, Health & Christianity", *Contact* 14, Christian Medical Commission, Geneva.
2. Jansen, G. *The Doctor-Patient Relationship in an African Tribal Society*, Van Gorcum & Co. BV, Assen, the Netherlands, 1973.
3. *Outreach*, 1975, **2** No. 16. Pub. Diocese of Owerri, PO Box 31, Owerri, Nigeria.
4. Idowu, Dr Bolaji. Quoted by Dr Stanley Lang, Link Letter, Dec 29 74, CMS, London.
5. Maclean, Una. *Magical Medicine*, Penguin, London, 1971.
6. *Outreach*, op cit
7. *Magical Medicine*, op cit p. 153.
8. Ibid p. 139, 141, 80.
9. *Health Care in China*, op cit. p. 96.
10. *Magical Medicine*, p. 112.
11. McCormick, James. *Journal of the Royal College of General Practitioners*, 1975, **25**, pp. 9–19.
12. Thomas, K. B. *British Medical Journal*, 1974, **1**, pp. 625–626.
13. Illich, Ivan, *Medical Nemesis*, Calder & Boyars, London, 1975, p. 21.
14. *The Times*, April 17 1973.
15. Mitchell, Robert C. *Witchcraft, Sin, Divine Power and Healing; the Aladura Churches and the Attainment of Life's Destiny among the Yoruba*, Christian Medical Commission, Geneva, 1968
16. *Magical Medicine*, p. 81.
17. Jansen, G. op cit. p. 34.
18. Sibisi, Harriet. "Some Aspects of Causality and Treatment of Disease", Seminar on Christianity in Post-Colonial Africa, May 9 1974, School of Oriental and African Studies, London.
19 Mitchell, Robert C. op. cit. p. 2.

Chapter 14

REVOLUTION OF LOVE?

"Did you know," said Joel to the pastor, in Joyce Peel's play *Valley of Decision*,[1] which exposes the corruption in a famine-stricken village, "that your Headmaster, who is also your church secretary, has sold six bags of milk powder on the black market instead of feeding it to his children?"

"I heard talk," replies Pastor Jebamani, "but I don't like to believe evil of my flock . . . I confine my interests to spiritual matters, Mr. Joel. . .". And as Joel presses him to act to redress other injustices, he counters: "You are young, Mr. Joel, young and impractical. The Church cannot take a moral stand in matters of politics and economics. God sent this famine, Mr. Joel; not these men." "You talk as if God sent the famine deliberately," cries out Joel. "These things are ingrained in the natural order. When they burst upon us, man has to choose whether to make them worse with his selfish greed and cowardice, or to join together and overcome them with courage and faith." But the pastor still objects and Joel's last words are "I'll leave you to your unspecific sermons . . . *I* can't separate religion from daily life."

Joyce brings the Minor Prophets up-to-date with burning earnestness, and as she writes one hears Amos crying "I hate your feasts . . . your solemn assemblies . . . let justice roll down like waters, and righteousness like an overflowing stream," and bursting out against those who are "trampling upon the needy, and . . . buying the needy for a pair of sandals."[2]

The same passion for justice fills Yohan Devananda,[3] Christian poet of Sri Lanka, of whom Bishop John Taylor has written so movingly.[4] He describes Yohan as "a gentle, Christ-like person, warm but a little withdrawn," an Anglican minister whose concern for the sorrows of his country has led him on into the field of social reflection and action. He saw the widening gulf between rich and poor, the plight of those working on the tea-plantations for tiny wages, and the need for a new society based on true justice for all, in which the Church would work selflessly for the 60% of school-leavers who could not find jobs.

He planned a farm in which all who joined it would share both in the work, and in the management and the profits. But just before the scheme began a rebellion of jobless young people broke out, only to be put down with the greatest severity.

Yohan wrote a poem of passionate feeling but also of balanced thought, in which he indicts influential groups which have contributed each in turn to the injustice, and among them:

. . . "religious leaders"—who
. . . "talk endlessly, mouthing empty phrases . . .

But they are silent and inactive
on the things that really matter,
social change, land reform, employment,
human relationships, human dignity,
involvement with the people."

He goes on, in deep earnestness:

"Radical changes are necessary,
structural changes,
revolution,
land reform, collective farms, reformed co-operatives,
changes in ownership, management, and production,
not merely in distribution,
also changes in worship and preaching,
in teaching and learning,
changes that will bring about new relationships between people,
new attitudes,
changes that will enable people to be people,
not merely animals,
not merely things, instruments or pawns,
changes that will make possible
a new society, a new man,
a new heaven, a new earth."

In many countries of the world today it seems that the lack of these very changes holds back any hope of adequate health care for those who need it most.

Trapped in Injustice

R. Jeffery[5] has described the pattern in one country in which the best medical care is available in the towns, the places where 75% of the doctors live. But as he says, it is the army, the senior civil servants and the large landowners who receive this high-grade care. The medical profession protects its own interests, choosing where its members will work, and resisting the use of auxiliaries. Prevention of disease is given lip service, but rural areas are relatively neglected. How could such a highly unequal health system ever be completely changed? It would be resisted strongly by the élite and the power groups.

Just allocation of land is essential for a healthy community, and in Pakistan President Bhutto has courageously decreed that no farmer may own more than 150 acres of irrigated land, and 300 unirrigated acres.[6] But it is easy for a landowner to distribute his holding between the members of his family, including small children, and the landless peasant and sharecropper remains as badly off as ever.

In Bangladesh it is the same: rural co-operatives are essential. But when a land-owning family forms itself into a co-operative, it still controls land, monopolizes government loans, exploits the small man and the co-operative becomes rural capitalism in disguise.[7]

It is hard to see how communities can be really healthy when they are trapped in such a situation, in a network of low wages, poor housing, insufficient food and unequal land tenure.

What we need is a radical change

"A girl in an office," writes Paul Gallet[8] (pen-name of a young French priest in South America), "earns about 5½ dollars a month (£2.75). Do you know what a working man earns here?" he continues. "Well under a dollar (50p) a day, on which to keep his wife and children." Even by 1963 standards these are tiny sums.

Paul is a buoyant soul who sings and dances along the road as he joins in a procession which is letting off fire-crackers. And he exults in "the joy of belonging to Christ forever . . . and of a heart that grows younger every day."

But when he thinks of life around him in Brazil, it tears at his whole being. "The average life expectancy," he reflects, "is twenty-seven years. When you are told that someone here is thirty, you think of him as old. In working-class districts cooking oil is sold not by the bottle but by the spoonful, and cigarettes are sold singly."

In the rickety houses built on stilts in the mud where he lives, there is illness everywhere. TB is rampant. "Hermogenes, spitting blood and dying of TB, had to stay in a miserable palm-leaf hut open to all the winds—the doctor refused to have him in hospital. We went to the sanatorium. I said 'He simply can't go home.' The matron agreed. But I had scarcely left when they turned him out again. But we still fought on. The neighbours made a real chain of love around him. And now—Hermogenes is a different man. He's looking for work. Everything says it's a miracle: a miracle of love."

As Paul meditates on these things, he burns with the longing to set forward "the defence of human dignity and humanity itself, and the fight for justice and respect for the poor."

He listens to the story of Francisco, a character in a story which is the story of all poor labourers in that part of the country. Francisco is in torment because his family is so hungry, and they haven't got a roof over their heads. The landowner gives him land, but in return insists on taking half the crop. The rest of the future harvest of rice has to be sold in advance, far below the fair price, as Francisco needs money desperately to improve his land. The landowner's cattle keep getting into his land, and destroying his crops. . . .

At length he joins with friends so that they can help each other. The farmers improve the roads, pay a teacher for the children, support each other. . . .

José, living in his beaten-earth hut, a few feet from the mud on the sea-shore, has the same vision of team work for progress, and leads his community in many improvements brought about by ACO, the Catholic workers association. "The neighbours know from experience that it has been the leaven of the gospel that has underlain these improvements," asserts Paul Gallet. And he goes on to urge, "What we need is a radical change in structures and in outlook. The revolution the Third World needs is a revolution of love. Everyone is convinced that revolution is bound to come. And who will make a revolution of love if it isn't Christians?" Over the door of the hut where he lives, tiny, fragile, made of wood and at the mercy of all the winds of heaven, are the words of Mauriac: "The moment your heart stops burning with love, those beside you will die of cold."

What the West eats

But deeply as we in the West may want to enter into the sorrows and struggles of the Third World, our urgent task is to see again to what extent *we* are responsible for the injustices and imbalances which exist there. The world food situation is now a well-known illustration of such imbalance.

The Food and Agriculture Organization of the United Nations estimates that 400 million people in the world are underfed.[9] This is a figure that is indeed quite impossible for us to grasp.

But it is not only these huge numbers which stagger us. It is the realization that malnutrition gravely lowers the resistance of small children to infections that makes the situation still more serious.

Meanwhile, as we now know well, Western Europe and North America are eating far too much—and eating it in such a wasteful way.

The rich one-third of the world eats half of all the cereals grown—one ton of cereal a year for each person in North America. But 60 to 90% of this is fed to cattle, 4 lbs. of grain being used to produce 1 lb. of meat. The United Kingdom produces 4·8 million tons of wheat a year, almost enough for its direct human needs. But it imports another 3·6 million tons, mostly for feeding cattle. Meanwhile, in the poor two-thirds of the world, the average daily calorie intake is 1,900 as against 3,100 in the West.

The Green Revolution in Asia held out great hopes that Asian countries could grow enough cereal for their needs, but plenty of fertiliser is needed for success, and the industrial countries take so much. They used 60·7 million tons in 1973, as against 16·8 million tons used in the poor countries with more than twice the population. The United States is estimated to use more fertiliser on lawns, golf courses and cemeteries than is used in the whole of India.[10]

Again, each Western European eats nearly twice as much protein every day as the average man in the Far East and Africa. And in Peru children starve from protein lack, while the Peruvian Government exports anchovies to feed cattle in North America.

In 1975 a new "International Soya Bean Futures Market" was opened in London. Soya contains 40% protein, and is one of the chief answers to the protein needs of the Third World. It ought to be good news that the United States is planting 1 out of every 6·5 arable acres with soya. But the whole emphasis in the new Market is on its value for animal foodstuffs, primarily to feed the West.[11]

By contrast, in Cuba the whole population shares equally in the distribution of protein and calories. Supplies of fish, milk and meat are not boosted up for export but used to improve the country's nutrition. Partly as a result of this, infant mortality is down to 27 per 1,000 live births, very nearly approaching the figure in Britain.[12]

Not only is food consumption so unfair, but so are both the distribution of other resources and the world's trading patterns. It seems a shame to keep instancing the United States, a country so generous in many ways, but yet with only 5·6% of the world's population it uses 40% of the world's raw materials. And its influence on world trade, together with the influence of Europe, is a life-and-death matter for the economy of so many nations.

Lord Caradon is a notable challenger of the attitude of the West to the just demands of developing countries. He quotes Jennifer Whitaker, assistant editor of America's *Foreign Affairs*, as saying "We (the United States) are on the wrong side of virtually every political issue vis-à-vis most of the Third World (which is most of the United Nations); on the Middle East; on Indo-China; on South Africa; on Portugal (before the coup); on Chile (since the coup). We are the chief upholders of international capitalism and as such the chief symbol of Western exploitation and Third World dependence."[13]

In desperate straits

Unhappily the United Kingdom does not show up in any better colours. When delegates from more than 100 developing nations met in 1975 at Lima, with its grim memories of Pizarro and the Conquistadores, for the Second General Conference of the UN Industrial Development Organization (UNIDO), they spoke of the injustice of the economic order in which they were trapped. Their countries had 70% of the world's population and 7% of its industrial output.

These nations have to spend scarce foreign exchange in buying industrial products from the developed world. But with aid going down to only 0·30 per cent of the donor countries' GNP (Gross National Product) in 1973: debts multiplying: oil prices quintupling since 1970: and the value of their raw materials falling steadily, while the cost of imported manufactured goods rises, they are in desperate straits. And where are the jobs needed for their 300 million unemployed and underemployed?

At this UNIDO conference the Group of 77, the loose working party of 104 developing countries, asked for big changes in the world's economic order. They spelt out their proposals, which included opening the markets of the developed nations to Third World products: rescheduling their debts: being brought into consultation over a reform of the international monetary system: allotting industries like textile manufacture to the poorer countries: and controlling "the unacceptable practices of the multinational corporations" such as ITT.

81 nations voted in favour, one against (the United States) and seven abstained, including Britain, whose delegation described the proposals as "almost totally unacceptable" to Western countries.[14]

It is true that at Lomé in February 1975, the EEC (European Economic Community) Conference, in which Britain played an important part, decided to give free access to the Community market for all manufactures from the 46 African, Caribbean and Pacific states represented there, and this is a major advance. In addition, provision was made to stabilise future prices of coffee, cotton, sisal and tea. But these 46 countries only represent 12% of the people of the Third World, and India and Bangladesh, with their population pressures and problems of poverty, are not yet included.[15] Moreover at that time the other essential changes demanded in Lima had not yet been met.

To quote Yohan Devananda again:

> "The struggle for emancipation is going forward.
> We have to mould our society accordingly,
> patiently,
> with invincible hope.
> We have to go forward—
> from a society that is still based
> largely on violence and competition
> . . . to a society that will be based
> essentially on community . . .
> taking account of all realities,
> both good and evil."

And who will make a revolution of love if it isn't Christians? But the time in which to make such peaceful change is short indeed.

References **Chapter 14**

1. "Valley of Decision", in *Voices of Revolution*, Joyce Peel, CLS Madras, 1971.
2. *Amos* 5. 21–24, 8. 4–6.
3. Devananda, Sevaka Yohan. *Violent Lanka*, 1973, CMS, London.
4. *CMS Newsletter*, No. 375, November 1973.
5. Jeffery, R. Appropriate Technology Conference, University of Edinburgh, September 1973, Section of Medicine (mimeo report).
6. *The Times*, March 2 1972.
7. Report of Savar Health Centre, No. 4, July 1973–April 1974. Gonoshasthya Kendra, PO Nayarhat, District Dacca, Bangladesh.
8. Gallet, Paul. *Freedom to Starve*, Penguin, London, 1972.
9. *The Guardian*, July 12 1974.
10. Report on World Food Conference, *New Internationalist,* November 1974.
11. *The Times*, April 3 1975.
12. "Cuba"; *World Health*, April 1975.
13. *The Guardian*, December 30 1974.
14. ibid April 1 1975.
15 *Comment*, CIIR, London, No. 25, 1975.

Chapter 15

IS IT ALL ANY GOOD?

Field Marshal Auchinleck, when lecturing once on "The Art of War", described a battle as a very rough and lawless game of football in which time after time the rules were broken, plans were thwarted, and the team's aims frustrated and wrecked.

Schemes of better health care appear to suffer in the same way. A new pattern is worked out, with what seems to be great benefits for those who are poorest and most needy. And then there is a sudden change of Government, an economic crisis, even an outbreak of fighting. And all new plans have to be shelved, and existing work may be slowed up or stopped.

Or corruption, which occurs of course in every country in the world, may mean that grants of money, drugs and food supplies just do not find their way to the places where they are needed most. In some countries family-planning campaigns seem to be failing to slow down population growth in spite of great efforts, food reserves have become dangerously low, efforts at reform of land tenure meet with great difficulties, medical education is not being adapted to meet national needs, and the control of diseases such as leprosy and bilharzia (schistosomiasis) appears harder than ever before.

Faced with such difficulties it is not surprising that medical workers in developing countries are often tempted to despair. The very size of the problems is overwhelming—so many hundreds of millions malnourished, such doubling of populations within one generation.

And the prophets of doom are many. Heilbroner, writing on the "*Human Prospect*", sees nothing but rapid population growth, war, and environmental collapse, with no hope of avoiding ultimate catastrophe.[1]

Hamburger draws an equally sombre picture, and glooms over the failure of nations to co-operate in meeting urgent ecological problems.[2] And Pearce Wright reminds us on the 30th anniversary of the Hiroshima atomic bomb that the nuclear powers have many times the destructive might needed to wipe out all life from the earth.[3]

In response to these solemn trends and warnings there are several things to be said.

Firstly it may indeed happen that Christians will have to share painfully in the difficulties and failures which others meet. A Christian leader referred recently to a country reeling under the combined blows of war, famine, flooding, corruption and population pressure. "Maybe everything will go down in chaos," he said. "But if so, I think that Christians should be there to go down with all the rest." True as this may be, it is a very terrifying prospect.

Where the difficulties are not so great, we should be clear about our role and our aims in medical work. Christians cannot provide more than a tiny fraction of the health care that a nation needs. But they ought to provide an example, a small working model, of what human living and caring can be like. Hakan Hellberg, a wise Finnish doctor, reminds us that "being significant" means "making a sign." We are a signpost pointing the way, or a candle trying to keep alight in dark times.

And we should not underestimate the value of such small enterprises, or the work of individual people. They can have wide and lasting effects.

Consider John Woolman, gentle American Quaker, who had a "tenderness towards all creatures", which extended most of all to the slaves whom he saw all around him, but also to cabin-boys in the miserable conditions of the tiny North Atlantic packet-boats, and to post-boys freezing to death as they worked the mail-coaches of 18th-century England.

He died of smallpox at York in 1772, lonely and often misunderstood. But his life and writings greatly influenced Jean Pierre Brissot of France, whose work led to the emancipation of the slaves in Haiti. He deeply impressed Clarkson, staunch worker with Wilberforce in abolishing Britain's slave trade. And he inspired Stephen Grellet, who in turn moved Alexander I of Russia to begin the abolition of serfdom, a reform carried out by his son Alexander II.[4]

Of John Lettsom, another Quaker, distinguished London physician, founder of the Royal Humane Society to save lives from drowning, and active in many other philanthropies, a medical historian has recently written "It would be hard to find anyone on record who so devoted his whole life, with sound and lasting effects, to what he could do himself, and stimulate public opinion to do, for the good of his fellow men."[5]

And in Georgina Battiscombe's deeply perceptive biography of Lord Shaftesbury she concludes, after speaking of the effect produced by his concern over "drains and dung-heaps, overcrowding, infection and water-supply," with the words "No man has ever done more to lessen the extent of human misery or to add to the sum of human happiness."[6]

So we can take heart, and believe that single lives, and much smaller undertakings than those I have mentioned, can be used by the Lord in His great purposes.

And most important of all, Christian health care is in obedience to the Lord's command that by love we should serve one another. Those who undertake it want to hear the Lord saying one day "Come, O blessed of my Father, inherit the kingdom prepared for you. . . . I was hungry and you gave me food, . . . I was sick and you visited me. . . ."[7] Maybe the schemes of health caring will fail to achieve all that was hoped; but a Christian is not interested in success as much as in being faithful, nor in achievement as much as in pleasing his Master.

And best of all, the Christian believes, against all appearances, that the world is not indeed going to end in atomic desolation, or total ecological disaster. Great difficulties and hardships lie ahead, but God is on the throne, and one day the Lord Jesus will return to take control.

Timothy Dudley-Smith sings:

"As I read the Gospel story
We shall see the Lord in glory,
We shall see the Lord in glory when He comes!"[8]

and so we shall, unless we have met Him in heaven beforehand. History is moving towards the time when everything will be put under His feet.

This was Shaftesbury's main incentive (which puzzled Georgina Battiscombe very greatly) and it urged him on to make the most of whatever time he had. He knew, as we know, that the small fragments of the Kingdom which are being built now will one day be part of a brilliant whole, when all wrongs are righted and all oppression ceases.

So it is indeed worth while, more than ever worth while, to meet human need where it is greatest, and to do it for Christ's sake.

References **Chapter 15**

1. Heilbroner, *The Human Prospect*, reviewed in *New Internationalist*, November 1974.
2. Hamburger J. "Future of man", *World Health*, September 1974.
3. *The Times*, August 6 1975.
4. Whittier, J. G. *Journal of John Woolman*, Smeal, Glasgow, 1882.
5. Newsom, C. *British Medical Journal*, 1975, **2**, pp. 382–383.
6. Battiscombe, Georgina. *Lord Shaftesbury, a Biography of the 7th Earl*, Constable, London, 1974.
7. *St. Matthew* 25. 34–36.
8. *Keswick Praise* (hymnbook of Keswick Convention) no. 269.

EPILOGUE

UNANSWERED QUESTIONS

Will the opportunities for witnessing to the love of Jesus be as great in community health projects as they were in the institution?

The answer is, I believe, that practical loving caring is itself a powerful Christian witness, wherever it is given. Like education, such care should enrich the whole of a man's personality and deepen his relationships with his family and neighbours. It stands by itself as a practical demonstration of love.

Commending the Lord Jesus by our words is something that we are to do everywhere, and may be more effective in the natural surroundings of a rural community, as delegates to a recent Nigerian health conference thought, than in the unfamiliar and often very busy setting of a hospital.[1]

What about the economics of such health care? How is it to be paid for? It is often said that patients will pay for curative treatment, but community health programmes cannot possibly be self-supporting.

This is a very difficult problem, which really deserves much fuller analysis than I feel able to give. Much that is written about community health today seems to be with national governments in mind. It is tacitly assumed that governments will pay for the health centres or senior medical auxiliaries, and will do so willingly, because the benefits are so substantial in relation to costs.

But Christian health enterprises have to raise funds some other way, and how are they to do this? Let it be said at first that no hospitals pay for themselves today except those of a nursing-home type which charge very high fees. And in community health work at least the sum involved can be kept smaller.

But still these sums of money have to be found, and those who need help most are the least able to pay.

The Aroles insisted that villagers who asked for curative treatment should pay for it. At Savar they established a family insurance scheme, not without difficulty. And John Sibley, though realizing that he had not got the complete answer, was thinking in terms of a medical insurance at Kojedo, with discount rates offered to the poorest 20% of the population.

Governments, central or local, may be willing to give grants. And then it seems reasonable that just as the world's problems of trade and development can only be solved if the richer countries give generous help, so the Church throughout the world should share the cost of new health ventures in developing countries, so long as the self-reliance and powers of decision of those on the spot are not undermined.

And every effort is needed to keep costs down by encouraging voluntary help, freely given in varied ways, and by fostering co-operation with traditional healers and the use of traditional herbal remedies.

These suggestions do not however provide a complete answer, and further study of the finance of small health schemes is greatly needed.

In conclusion, Christian concern for health is surely something different from providing basic health care for a community, at however simple a level. It is rather an attitude of mind, a desire to turn love into practical action, an earnest wish for the happiness of families other than our own, a recognition of the great potential of children and their mothers, an urge to see man's dignity recognized and acknowledged, irrespective of race, social position, mental handicap or whatever.

And does it not reach out to include deep sympathy for those with fears and anxieties—so similar to the anxieties we experience ourselves—and a burning desire for justice for those who suffer ill-health, hunger and poverty?

If Christian health care is all this and more, and done in the spirit of the Lord Jesus, then it will be varied and "untidy", a new scheme here and a fresh project there, a bubbling-up of human-ness and humility and compassion and unselfish giving in all sorts of places, a partnership of layman with professional, a living growing plant, mainly very simple in appearance, but with its seeds carried to places of research, teaching and national planning.

It will change its form as new needs arise, but will continue to bear fruits of increased human happiness and strengthened inner resources, all in loving dependence on the One who can make all things new.

References

Epilogue

1. Report on a Workshop on Community Health, Jos, June 1975, Christian Health Association of Nigeria, Lagos.

UPPSALA 68

On the Bread of Heaven I long to feed,
The cry of my soul is—Jesus!
'Tis the Living Water alone I need,
My heart is athirst for Jesus.
There's none other's blood that can cleanse my sin:
No other guest dare I welcome in:
How else can my spirit to heaven win?
I crave for Yourself, Lord Jesus.

'Gainst poverty, ignorance we shall fight,
But the need of the world is Jesus.
And sickness, oppression—let's break their might:
Yet still our heart's call is—Jesus!
Justice and dignity we must gain
For our brother man, and break ev'ry chain
So that full human life we may all obtain,
But O, we want You, Lord Jesus!

Index

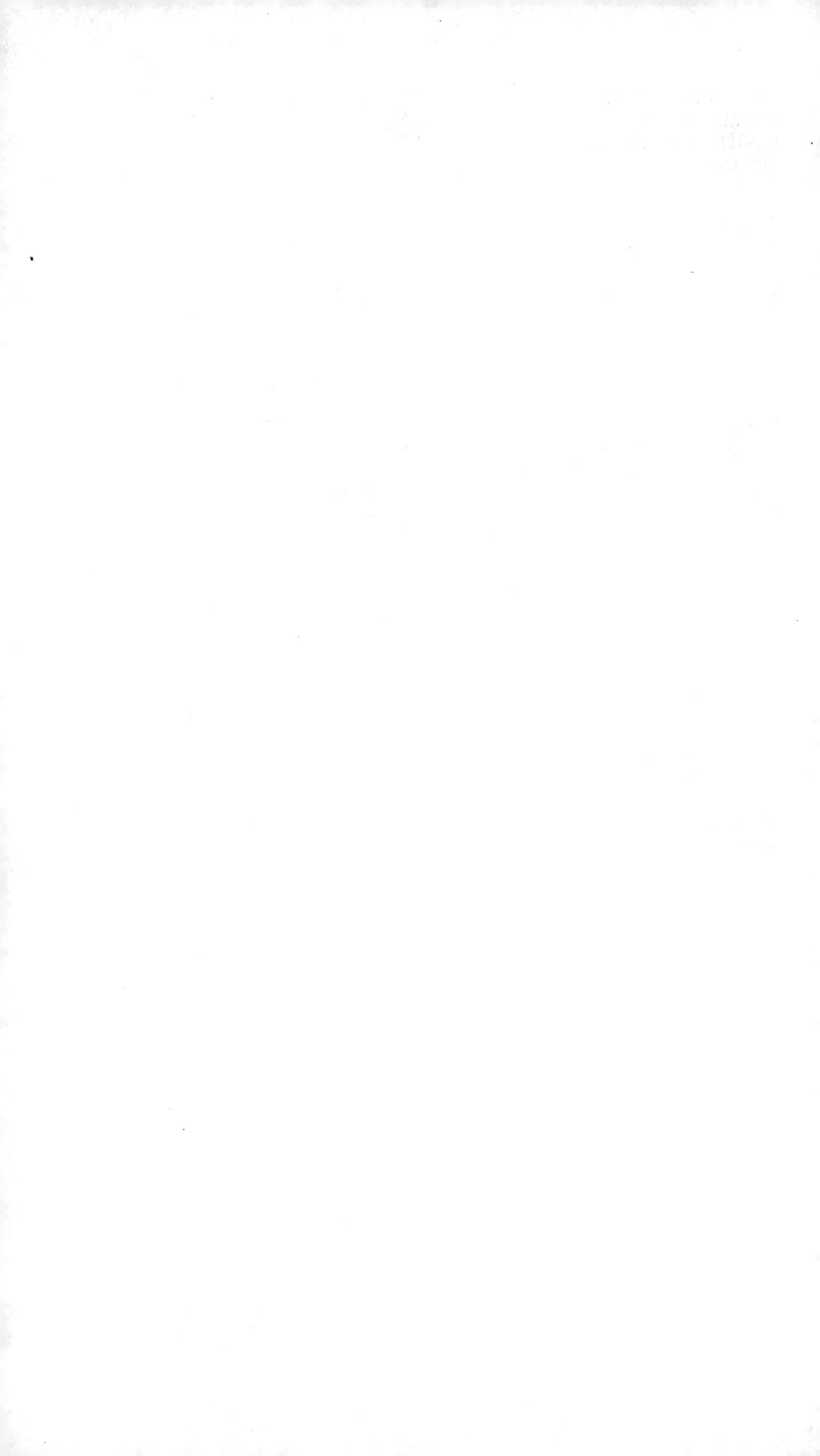